PRAISE FOR
CHRONIC RESILIENCE

"Danea Horn has put an honest and wise voice to the intimate journey of illness. She lights a fire for self-compassion and puts stress in its place, while providing empowering suggestions for living with grace and *Chronic Resilience*. I highly recommend this groundbreaking book."

> —KRIS CARR, *New York Times* bestselling
> author of *Crazy Sexy Diet*

"I highly recommend *Chronic Resilience*, not only to those who suffer from chronic illness but to those who love them. Danea Horn promises that her book will help the chronically ill become caregivers to themselves, and she delivers— magnificently. People with chronic illness need concrete tools for learning how to live with grace and purpose despite their difficult circumstances. This book offers those tools. It describes in detail ten practical guidelines for managing the stress and challenges of illness. Exercises are included so that readers can make each guideline their own and learn to incorporate it into their everyday lives. In addition, Ms. Horn not only shares her personal experiences working with these practical tools (which feels like chatting with an old friend), but also includes intimate conversations with nine other women who suffer from chronic illness. This book will help you transform the stress of chronic illness into a life of acceptance, purpose, and gratitude. It's a gem."

> —Toni Bernhard, author of *How to Be
> Sick: A Buddhist-Inspired Guide for the
> Chronically Ill and Their Caregivers*

"Danea provides an invaluable perspective on how to be resilient when battling a chronic illness. A must read to help you navigate the emotions successfully."

—Lori Hartwell, author of *Chronically Happy: Joyful Living in Spite of a Chronic Illness*

"I love this book. It is funny, touching, and true. *Chronic Resilience* is a best friend for anyone impacted by chronic illness. Intimate and authentic, tender and wise, Danea offers everyone the benefit of her courageous triumph . . . a life well lived . . . debilitating diseases be danged!"

—Penelope Young Andrade, LCSW, author of *Emotional Medicine Rx: Cry When You're Sad, Stop When You're Done, Feel Good Fast*

Chronic
Resilience

10} Sanity-Saving Strategies
for Women Coping with
the Stress of Illness

Danea Horn, CPC

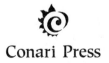

Conari Press

First published in 2013 by Conari Press, an imprint of
Red Wheel/Weiser, LLC
With offices at:
665 Third Street, Suite 400
San Francisco, CA 94107
www.redwheelweiser.com

Library of Congress Cataloging-in-Publication Data
Horn, Danea.
    Chronic resilience: 10 sanity-saving strategies for women coping with the
stress of illness / Danea Horn, CPC.
        pages cm
    Summary: "Chronic illness comes with stress, and Chronic Resilience pro-
vides a complete self-help blueprint for managing the difficulties chronic illness presents. Certified life coach and speaker Danea Horn, who suffers from
chronic kidney disease, infertility, and other demanding health challenges due
to a birth disorder, offers techniques and ways to rebound from the pressures
of having a body that's doing things you wish you could control.Chronic Resilience shows how to: Stop pushing yourself so hard. Use research to empower -
not frighten - yourself. Let yourself be pissed! Train your troops in how to care
for you. Cultivate focus and flexibility. Find things to be grateful for. Focus on
what you can do, not what you can't. Each chapter also contains highlights of
interviews with women dealing with chronic health issues ranging from cancer
to organ transplant, Crohn's disease, rheumatoid arthritis (RA), MS, Cushing's
disease, diabetes, and others"-- Provided by publisher.
    Summary: "Chronic Resilience provides a complete self-help blueprint for
having a good life while managing the difficulties every chronic illness presents"—Provided by publisher.
    ISBN 978-1-57324-594-4 (pbk.)
    1. Women—Mental health—Popular works. 2. Women—Diseases—Popular
works. 3. Chronic diseases—Popular works. 4. Self-care, Health—Popular
works. I. Title.

    RC451.4.W6H668 2013
    616'.044082—dc23

                                    2013000160

Cover design by Nita Ybarra
Interior by Maureen Forys, Happenstance Type-O-Rama

Printed in Canada
F

10 9 8 7 6 5 4 3 2 1

The paper used in this publication meets the minimum requirements of the
American National Standard for Information Sciences—Permanence of Paper
for Printed Library Materials Z39.48-1992 (R1997).

For Phillip
Love is deep, sweet and strong.

CONTENTS

ACKNOWLEDGMENTS

My deepest gratitude to Meredith Israel Thomas, Sarah Ramey, Charity Tillemann-Dick, Lauren Nastasi, Kelly Young, Nicole Lemelle, Sharmyn McGraw, Sandra Joseph, and Mari Ruddy, my warrior sisters who contributed their chronic resilience. Your stories, honesty, and grace made a profound impact on the book and my life. I am a better patient because of each of you.

To my editor Caroline Pincus, your commitment and enthusiasm were essential ingredients in creating this book. You have been an absolute joy to work with. I appreciate everyone at Red Wheel/Weiser immensely for your dedication and guidance. A special thank you to Jan Johnson for your interest, encouragement, and introducing me to Caroline.

Dr. Danielle Vecchio, my pediatrician. Thank you for being there to welcome me into the world and to care so compassionately for my health. You have always been an integral piece of my family's life and we love you.

To Dr. Hardy Hendren and the other doctors and nurses who have cared for me. The passion and concern you have for your patients is evident in so many ways. You made me whole and I am so thankful.

To Trisha Sterling, you are my saving grace. The generosity you offered to a new friend helped bring my book to life.

Thank you to Lee and Shayne Fischer, my in-laws. Your support has been a cherished part of the writing process.

To Feroshia Knight, my friend and mentor. Thank you for the education you blessed me with and for your steadfast belief in my potential as a coach and game-changer.

Mahogany Mañalac, Kelly Taylor, Kelly Hoffman, and Carolyn Cuozzo, your friendship has made it possible to accomplish more than I could have dreamed of. Thank you for the phone calls, brunches, notes, late nights, and welcoming hugs. You have my heart.

To my in-laws, Bob and Cheryl Burquist, I feel incredibly blessed to have you as family. Cheryl, I cherish our relationship. I am so thankful for your love and mothering of me.

John Foos, Dad, my biggest fan. Thank you for always seeing the light in me, especially when I'm struggling to find it myself. You have taught me to love in spontaneous and compassionate ways. The tug on my heart toward the mountains is there because of you, and I am so grateful for that.

Marilyn Joy, Mom, my kindred spirit. You embody the love only a mother can. At 10,000 feet alone with your two year old, your strength became my resilience. Thank you for your devotion as a caregiver, mother, and friend. You continually demonstrate selfless kindness in ways I can only aspire to. I am immeasurably blessed to be your daughter.

Abbey and Emma, my fuzzy girls. I appreciate your company and patience during the writing process. Your sweet faces and waggy tails have brought boundless joy into my life.

To my incredible husband, Phillip. Thank you for your unwavering support and the freedom to pursue my life's work. You have demonstrated unconditional love in ways that have amazed and healed me. I am grateful for you and our life together each day.

INTRODUCTION

When I was in eighth grade, a few girls started a rumor that I was stuck up. They came to this conclusion because I stand with my left leg slightly bent, and apparently that is the universal symbol for stuck up. Did you know this?

I promise you I'm friendly. My "snooty teen" stance is one of the only visible clues to my diagnosis. The other thing you might notice is that the top joint in each of my thumbs doesn't bend. It's my party trick the school-yard kids found endlessly fascinating. My fourth grade teacher, on the other hand, was not amused as she struggled to get me to hold my pencil the way other students did during cursive lessons.

Diagnosis

While these two trivial quirks seem unrelated, they are connected by a disorder my doctor once called "nature's worst malformation." I was born with VACTERL Association, an acronym which stands for the different parts of the body it may affect: *V* for vertebral, *A* for anal, *C* for cardiovascular, *T* for tracheal, *E* for esophageal, *R* for renal (kidney), and *L* for limb. A child has VACTERL Association if she has a malformation in three or more of the systems listed. Piece by piece, my puzzle eventually included all of the letters except for *C*, cardiovascular.

In addition to the thumb thing, here's a rundown of the way VACTERL manifested in my body: my left hip was dislocated, and my spine has some malformed vertebrae and a slight "s" curve, scoliosis. My reproductive organs, bowel, and urethra were jumbled into a single opening. I have a double uterus. My trachea and esophagus were not properly connected to each other or my stomach. My left kidney was missing, and my right kidney had anatomical defects. Lastly, my left arm and left fingers are slightly underdeveloped and are shorter than on my right side.

I am very fortunate to have been born when I was because medicine had advanced to the level my body demanded. Before I was two years old I'd had ten reconstructive surgeries to put things back into proper working order. Growing up, I endured choking incidents due to the anomalies in my esophagus, pneumonia hospitalizations, experimentation with diet and medication to create a healthy digestive system, and countless doctor visits and tests to monitor the development of my spine and the function of my single kidney.

As the years passed, my family took a collective sigh of relief as it seemed that my health was stable and we were through the worst of it. While I am exceptionally fortunate to be where I am with the start I had, my healing journey continued longer than we hoped. You'll read about the details of the path I've walked throughout the book, but I want to let you know where I'm at today.

I am currently on the national kidney transplant waiting list. I was hopeful that my body would hold off on needing a transplant until science caught up and I could grow my own new kidney in a petri dish, but it doesn't look promising. The doctors believe I have enough function to last a few more years as my name creeps its way toward the top of the list.

My back gets painfully tired quickly, and I have muscle spasms every six months or so. I also have decreased lung capacity from the anomalies in my trachea and esophagus that mimics untreatable asthma. You won't see me running a marathon, or more than two blocks, anytime soon. Because of my decreased kidney function and two smaller uteruses instead of one large one, pregnancy is not in my future. If you've dealt with infertility as part of your illness, chapter 10 talks more about my experience with this.

I have been married to Phillip, the love of my life, for ten years. We have moved several times since we've been married, and I mention that a few times as you read along. The succession of our moves is as follows: two years in Colorado, two years in Southern California, four years in Portland, and we're going on three years in Northern California. We live with our furry kids, Abbey and Emma, terrier rescues who bring us joy each day.

Learning from Illness

When the girls spread the "stuck-up" rumor about me in middle school, I wasn't upset. I wasn't embarrassed. And I didn't try to stand differently to blend in, because I knew that the rumor said more about them than it did about me. My abnormal reaction, for an insecure adolescent, is all credited to my parents.

My parents never ever made me feel cursed, burdened, or unlucky for my health challenges. In fact, I was raised to feel proud of what I had been through. They were encouraged by the capacity of an infant to endure and heal from such tremendous obstacles. They welcomed the journey I was on and worked hard to give me the best chance to live as normal a life as possible.

As I grew up, I knew that if I could be strong and resilient coming out of my first surgery at one day old, then I always had capacity. I felt that my unusual path had a purpose in my life, and I accepted the obstacles wholeheartedly. With childlike faith, I bounded through my school years believing that my life and my body were just as they were supposed to be. But then came my twenties.

As my kidney function declined and I learned that pregnancy would not be safe, I had to give up things that I wanted. I became less accepting of my health. I started to think maybe I was cursed, burdened, or unlucky. Stress played a bigger role in my life and in my relationship with my body.

I read book after book about healing and the mind-body connection, and I was dismayed that I couldn't heal myself with prayer, meditation, or diet. I misguidedly took on the burden of feeling responsible for my illness. I thought that maybe I was too negative, or karma was following me around creating pain and loss. I shamed myself for the state of my health. It wasn't just that there was something wrong with my body, there was something wrong with me. My body didn't work correctly, and it was my fault. Talk about a burden!

By the time I ventured into my thirties, I was tired of this cycle and ready to develop a new relationship with myself. I reviewed my life and everything I knew about my health. I thought about my childhood, and the version of myself that was too young to feel guilty about getting sick. I saw that not only was she accepting of her body, she was accepting of her emotions and spirit, too. She had compassion for the bumps in the road. She'd cry when she was in pain and bounce on trampolines when she felt good. She wasn't ashamed of or frightened by her scars (both emotional and physical). She had lived what I needed to relearn. From the mirror I'd put up to my life came this book. I titled it *Chronic Resilience* because I realized that to be the essence of gracefully coping with illness. Life is not about figuring out how to be happy and get your way all the time. Instead, we are called to experience the rollercoaster that is life.

The Conversations

In addition to sharing experiences from my own life, in each chapter you will meet a unique and insightful woman coping with chronic illness. In chapter 3, Charity Sunshine Tillemann-Dick shares her story of recovering from not one but two double-lung transplants to reclaim her career as a world-renowned opera singer. Chapter 5 will introduce you to Kelly Young, a mother of five who has rheumatoid arthritis (RA). She shares how she adjusts her environment to accommodate RA while fostering her spiritual growth—a "side effect," she says, of chronic illness. You will meet Sharmyn McGraw in chapter 8. After seven years, and countless doctor appointments with no answers, she researched her way to a diagnosis of Cushing's disease, which had caused a one-year, one-hundred-plus–pound weight gain. In addition to these three amazing women, there are six more stories profiling: cancer, auto-immune-like disorders, idiopathic pulmonary hypertension, Crohn's disease, multiple sclerosis, and diabetes.

Each woman I interviewed was generous and honest. They shared the day-to-day struggles and triumphs of dealing with illness while living a full and productive life. They have not been miraculously cured. They have the same fears, frustrations, and hopes that you or I do. They have also learned quite a few things while navigating the rough waters of their diagnosis, and I am honored to bring you their wisdom. The conversations I had with these inspiring women were the most treasured part of putting this book together. Their words lit a path in my life, and I know they will do the same for you as you manage your diagnosis.

How to Read This Book

As we learn how to become resilient to the challenges and stress of chronic illness, I'll ask you to do more than simply read these pages. Changing your outlook and your life requires active participation, and there is some self-reflection I'd like you to do along the way.

Journaling

Throughout the book you will find journal exercises. I have journals everywhere. Some are green, some are brown, spiral-bound, and hardback. They hold deep, dark secrets, personal revelations, and my goals for the future. Some have specific functions: this one is for gratitude, that one is to vent. Others are a random mix. I highly encourage you to treat yourself to a new journal and pen. A book can be a bunch of words on a page, or it can be a catalyst to create something new. Open your journal when you see this symbol:

Read the exercise and then take a moment to apply it to your own life.

Embracing Chronic Resilience

Illness comes with stress—it's a package deal. In these pages I'll show you some ways to rebound from the pressures of having a body that's doing things you wish you could control. We'll explore techniques and philosophies that can help you become a more supportive caregiver to yourself so you can cry when you're in pain and bounce on trampolines when you feel good.

This book is an ownership tool. Each of the ten chapters presents a technique for managing the stress of illness that you can pull from to walk the journey you are on. Read through the book once, and then pick two or three chapters that resonate with you the most. Reread those with a focus on how you will apply the lessons to your own life. As time goes by you may feel prompted to revisit other chapters, but don't overwhelm yourself by trying to move a mountain all at once. Mountains are moved one rock at a time.

When I asked Charity (chapter 3) how her illness has changed her view of herself, she replied, "It confirmed my thoughts on my extreme specialness!" That is what I pray this book does in your life. Illness doesn't make you less special—it makes you *more* special.

OK, I know you are probably not feeling very special right now; you are probably frustrated, in pain, and dealing with annoying limitations. I'm not asking you to pretend that things are rosier than they are—illness *sucks*. It absolutely does. But you are strong and resilient. There are things you can do to make it manageable, and if you are honest, patient, and compassionate with yourself, these tools can help you feel just how extremely special you are. Trust me. You'll see.

CHAPTER 1

Take Ownership of
Your Wellness

Why on earth would I want to own a body that is broken? One that has aches and pains, needs medication, ruins plans, and embarrasses me? I would never buy it from a store, order it from a catalog, try to replicate it on my own, or borrow it from someone else. Still, when I wake up in the morning my body is there, ready to be moved through my day, to surprise me at any moment, and to make plans of its own without consulting me. My body is wild, unpredictable, rough around the edges, a pain in the ass (sometimes literally), but it is mine. This is the point that we start from: living with something that we did not choose or approve of.

One moment you're standing on the shore, the next you're swept up by the tide to bob and sway in a churning sea. Control, the one thing so desperately wanted, is lost in the swells. You kick and tread to be cured and supported. Kick and tread to dictate the future. Kick and tread in search of the shore. And then the sea reminds you of the depths you're dealing with and that it's time for a new strategy.

The *T* Word

My husband Phillip and I moved to Portland, Oregon, in 2006. At that time, I was monitoring my kidney function through blood tests every six months, so I made sure to find a nephrologist (kidney specialist) soon after we settled in. During my first checkup, my new doctor mentioned that he wanted me to establish a relationship with a urologist (urinary tract specialist) because he would be "on the transplant team." Everything came to a halt as I wondered, did he really just say the *T* word? In relation to *me?* I could only see the back of the doctor's white lab coat when he said it; he was typing the urology referral into the computer. I don't think he realized that this was the first time I had heard the world "transplant" in regard to my kidney. Up until that point, I assumed that my health as a spry twenty-something would mature into my being a spry sixty-something grandma; but apparently I was mistaken. I asked for clarification, and he replied that my level of kidney function would not last for the rest of my life and someday I would need a transplant.

A flood of fear washed over me. My view of my health suddenly changed from "I keep an eye on my kidney and take a few meds" to "I'm sick." Sick equaled scared. I left the doctor's office and walked through the dim parking garage back to my car, a flickering orange light illuminating the tears running down my face. Sob after sob, my situation closed in on me. My mind went through crude calculations of how many years it would be before I'd need a transplant, and who in my circle of friends and family was going to be the "lucky" one to donate a kidney. Alone in your car is not a good place to pull yourself together. Facts get fuzzy between the seat and the steering wheel. There is no passenger there to offer reason or a "we'll get through this" touch. There's only you, worrying that things are about to get really, really bad.

I was afraid to eat after that appointment. I didn't know if the thief who had taken my kidney function was hidden in the extra piece of pizza I was known to swipe.

What about the sugar in my lemonade? Or was coffee the culprit? How could something be happening in my body without my awareness or consent? I was supposed to be the guardian of my body, and somehow a burglar had slipped past me. I was determined to not let it happen again.

Up to this point in my life VACTERL had been a challenge, it had upset me and embarrassed me, but it wasn't anything I couldn't work around. There was just something extra dramatic about the idea that I would need someone else's organ put into my body to stay alive. That *T* word was making me tired and out of breath. I was confused and feeling victimized by my own body. In my angst, I sat and watched my power leave in the knapsack of the thief who had just changed my life.

Why Me?

Have you ever asked yourself, why me? Of all the people, and all the lifestyles, and all the everything, why *me?* You rack your brain for an answer: you think back to what you ate, what you stressed about, and all the snooze-alarm mornings when you only dreamt about the gym. You wonder if God is challenging you, and you question how strong you must be to face something so blatantly crappy.

"Why me?" has a thousand different answers. Philosophers, pastors, priests, revolutionaries, friends, even the random Facebook acquaintance all seem to have an opinion about why things come into our lives when they do and how. The theories run the gamut:

- "The Secret"—You attract your experiences based on your thoughts and feelings.

- "The Karma"—You are being punished.

- "The Guilt"—You are punishing yourself.

- "The Tough Love"—You are strong enough to handle it.

- "The Exorcist"—Disease is evil incarnate and has waged a war on your turf.

- "The Darwin"—It is just evolution, a random draw of the short straw.

- "The Hippie"—You are playing out an archetypal pattern to learn a lesson your soul needs.

- "The Mrs. Fields"—You are too stressed and ate too many cookies.

- "The Evangelical"—You do not have enough faith in God's healing power.

And the list goes on . . .

Most of the popular answers to "why me?" are ridiculous attempts to pull back the curtain and reveal the wizard, with little aim to provide comfort or understanding. "Why me?" is a complex question—it shows our innate desire to figure life out. Behind that two-word question is a yearning to control. If I could just figure out "why me?" then maybe I could fix what is broken and make things go back to how they were before.

Most often, we look outside ourselves for answers. I have spent many an afternoon sitting on the floor of the self-help section at the local Barnes & Noble, searching for the answer to that "why" question. A title will jump out, and I will think, "That's it! This book will tell me why my life is messed up and how I can magically fix it." When I read *The Power of Your Subconscious Mind* by Joseph Murphy, I thought that repeating positive thoughts was going to be the cure. After Eckhart Tolle's *The Power of Now*, I thought, "Oh, that's it. I wasn't living in the *now*. Once I fully live in the *now* everything will be perfect." I studied metaphysics, Christianity, and Buddhism. I searched my psyche for feelings and thoughts that needed to be healed. I prayed to increase my faith. I began to see my health as a manifestation of being separated from God, a belief in "dis-ease" that was harming my body. I became frustrated with myself and with my inability to channel healing love as I watched my lab results get worse. My initial question of "why" became a merry-go-round of questioning everything I thought I knew to be true. And so it went, book after book, until I had a bookcase filled top to bottom with answers, none of which seemed to miraculously fix what I envisioned as broken.

Years after I began my quest, I was driving from Sacramento toward the Sierra Nevada Mountains on Interstate 80. The city's crowded cement and flashy billboards had just left my rearview mirror. I took a deep breath and let my chest sink into the seat as my hands dropped from ten and two to four and six. My mind wandered to the great thinkers that lined my bookshelf. So many of them talk about the idea that we are spiritual beings. To heal and be prosperous, we have to connect with the spiritual side of ourselves, the side that is perfect and complete.

The spiritual journey is described much like my drive. The ego is the city, with its fight to be something. The neon advertisements and cement attempt to build up the prosperous but end up crowding out true beauty. Outside the city, the expanse is vast and peaceful. It is naturally beautiful. The trees don't need to try to be anything because they already are everything. I wondered why I wasn't like the trees yet. I had been studying for so long to get out of the city and into the trees, and I was frustrated with myself. The question arose, "why am I still dealing with the same crap I've been dealing with for years?" Then, without books or seminars or websites or coaches or any guru, an answer came.

The idea was so simple and so obvious you'll probably laugh that I didn't realize this sooner. I realized that *I am human*, and all of the cells in my body let out a collective sigh of relief.

Being Human

You are born completely dependent. You need to be fed, changed, cleaned, burped, and carried around. Each year you get a bit more independent: you take your first step, you dress yourself in hot pink tights and a green jumper, you hold hands at recess, you learn algebra, you terrify your parents by learning to drive, and eventually you fly from the nest. The gradual grasping of self-reliance gives you the idea that you have control over your life.

Illness laughs at this notion of control. We don't control everything that happens within our bodies because, as I so groundbreakingly discovered, we're human. Part of being human is experiencing pain, loss, stress, and heartache. It is the journey we all take. Each page I turned in all those books was a search for how to get out of being human. I had been looking for a spell that would prevent me from having to live through the tough stuff. I was pushing hard against something that wasn't going to go away.

Ownership

Imagine with me that you have moved into a new house and the moving crew put your 150-pound dresser on the wrong side of the bedroom. You wanted it to the right of the window, and they placed it to the left. You think, "I'll just move it myself," and you lean into the dresser, but it doesn't budge. You turn around, dig your heels into the carpet, and try pushing with your back, but that doesn't work either. Then you walk to the other side and pull with all of your might. The dresser is still to the left of the window, but now you are sweating and out of breath. That is stress.

The tension you put against the dresser is similar to the tension you place against illness. Illness is in your life for a conglomeration of reasons, and you can push with your front and push with your back, but it is still something you have to face.

Once you realize that the dresser is staying put, you decide to decorate around it. You no longer have to shove the dresser somewhere else. Tension is gone, and you can move on. The challenge is to figure out how to piece your life together around your diagnosis. The first step is to stop pushing so dang hard.

We push because illness just showed up. It feels like a misplaced tragedy from someone else's life. Like a bad Christmas gift, it doesn't match anything you own. It is unfair that you have to take responsibility for something you didn't choose. Yet, the circumstances of your life are yours to own. No matter what your diagnosis, you've got to go all in, with both feet, completely submerged.

It is important to claim ownership of your health because you already own it. You did not decide to get sick, but you live with your body every day. You are the one who has the intestines that like to play tricks, and you read blog after blog to learn how others shoot back apple cider vinegar and eat macrobiotics.

If you do not take ownership of your health, I can assure you that someone or something else will. Your emotions and thoughts will bounce around like ping-pong balls ricocheting off every opinion, study, test result, article, and sideways look you receive. The especially juicy, dramatic, and horrific thoughts tend to be the ones that we ruminate on. They also zap energy and impede healing. Not cool.

Becoming ill is a threat—to our lifestyle, and maybe even to our existence. When we feel threatened, it can be easy to cope by giving life the silent treatment. But, responsibility is paramount to every healing process. It is up to you to take on your wellness and live life as fully as possible. There is no person, book, seminar, or tweeted quote that can do this for you. You are being called to own your life.

The day I heard "transplant" for the first time, I wasn't only processing the idea of needing a kidney transplant, which would naturally involve some tears—I was feeding the drama of it. I was letting one word dictate how I was going to feel, mentally and physically. It took me a while to wake up to what I was doing. When my eyes were open, I saw that nothing had changed with my health except hearing the *T* word. Not my diet, not my exercise patterns. Nothing. Each time I felt out of breath or tired or in pain, I reminded myself of the health I still had and remembered the idea of needing a transplant was, at that point in my life, just one possibility for my future.

> It is up to you to take on your wellness and live life as fully as possible. There is no person, book, seminar, or tweeted quote that can do this for you.

A few more months passed, my fatigue decreased, and I was less scared of my own organs. When I was back at that same doctor's office for my next checkup, he changed his opinion and said, "who knows what's going to happen; your lab results have been stable every time I've seen you." I had a brief moment of triumph. I had been resilient. I had pulled up my big girl pants and pulled myself together. Problem solved! Or so I thought.

Ownership Is Not . . .

There is an important distinction to make here. Ownership does not mean that you "own" your disease. If you "own" your illness that probably means it has become your identity. When you begin to identify yourself as "a cancer patient" or say you "suffer from chronic fatigue" or "are a sick person with lupus," you give a level of importance to the disease—one it does not deserve.

It is completely understandable why we do this. As a society we connect through shared experiences of pain. It's what we gab about with our girlfriends, it's what gets us out of work, and let's face it, when you want your hubby to make dinner, a bit of whining about your aching back never hurt. Illness can cause love and attention to come your way that was otherwise hard to find. Identifying in this way and soaking in the benefits of being ill only keeps us in that pattern. Be honest with yourself about your relationship with your health and body. If you feel you have become entrenched in identifying with your diagnosis, seeing a therapist can help you change that pattern. We will discuss various healing professions in chapter 6.

Ownership is not merely acceptance. It is much bigger than that. Pretend you are on vacation in what is supposed to be gorgeous, sunny San Diego. Unfortunately, a wayward storm has come through, and now everything is all drippy. You can accept that your beach plans have been rained out and spend all weekend sulking in your hotel room watching reruns of *How I Met Your Mother*, or you can change your plans. Visit some of the amazing museums and restaurants in the city. Grab an umbrella and walk through Balboa Park anyway. Likewise, you can accept that you have been diagnosed with an illness and spend all day, every day in bed, or you can use that as a cue to adjust your plans. With acceptance comes the possibility of giving in and giving up.[1] You may not have resistance to your present reality, but there is no motivation to take action, either. People can let years go by like this, accepting, but also completely disengaged from, life, as if their illness has given them a Get Out of Life Free card.

Ownership Is . . .

What exactly *is* ownership? How do you take ownership?

Ownership is a decision to take responsibility for your life and your healing. It is that simple and that complex all at the same time. Make a decision to be open to the challenges that are already in your life. Going from clenched fist to open palm releases a lot of tension. Doing that frames every pain and annoyance in a way that makes it easier to deal with. Illness can be an invitation to become a deeper, stronger, wiser, more kick-ass you.

As you open to your experience, you will listen more to your body. It has a story to tell, and an owner learns to listen to her body carefully. When I have pushed myself too hard, my back gives me a gentle nudge that it has had enough. I can listen to that nudge and rest, or I can push harder and spend the next day on a heating pad on the couch. Rather than ignoring what hurts, allow your body a voice in your decisions and actions. This does not mean skipping yoga every time you're tired. Skilled owners can tell the difference between laziness and concerns that need attention. Listen to your body for a few weeks and you will be able to tell the difference between pains that need rest and pains that need to be moved through.

A few years after I first heard it mentioned, the *T* word came up again—this time at a different nephrologist's

---

1 Toni Bernhard, *How to Be Sick* (Massachusetts: Wisdom Publications, 2010), 81.

office, in a different city. I had created a nice illusion for myself. After the Portland doctor declared that I was stable, I assumed I wouldn't need to think about a transplant again. I felt healthy and had stopped obsessing. I was saying my affirmations and eating spinach and tofu. I had "drunk the Kool-Aid," had fully bought in—I was even giving speeches about attracting health through a positive attitude, for goodness' sake.

The same day as one of my presentations, two hours after leaving the podium, I learned that the kidney disease had progressed. The thief was back for more. The diagnosis had moved from stage 3 to stage 4 (kidney failure is stage 5), and the doctor was starting to float the idea of getting me on the transplant list. It was a blatant reminder that I was, in fact, not in control of this disease or my future. Although books and affirmations eased my symptoms and stress, they had not yet gotten me out of being human.

In an eerie déjà vu, I found myself back crying in my car. Our ride home from dinner that evening was an alarming premonition when NPR hosted an hour-long dialysis special to discuss the lifesaving treatment for patients in kidney failure. I pouted, sulked, ate cheesy pasta and loads of sugar, and whined to Phillip. I saw my mind heading back to that first parking garage with the flickering orange light where worry took hold.

A good night's sleep can change a lot, and by the next morning, I was determined to do things differently. This time, rather than indulge in a six-month pity party, I asked a question.

What Is in My Control?

Being a Harry Potter reader, I know that I'm a "muggle" (human). I didn't get to go to Hogwarts School of Witchcraft and Wizardry, and I don't have a magic wand to *presto-chango!* control my future, but there is a whole list of things in my control that can influence my response to that future. I can control my diet and exercise habits, and I can control what I focus on.

You take ownership by deciding what is in your control and placing laser-beam focus on that. Ownership is a bumpy ride with lots of twists and turns. As I did, you will be called to learn lessons over and over again—ones

> You take ownership by deciding what is in your control and placing laser-beam focus on that.

you thought you had already mastered. You will also get to decide over and over again to be an owner—to step up and claim the responsibility that is being asked of you. Knowing what is in your control gives you clarity about what your duties as an owner actually are.

After I asked, "What is in my control?" I put a plan together, and I refocused my thoughts and actions toward health. I began researching nutrition; I determined how many days of the week I would work out, and what exercises I would do. I did not give myself the luxury of contemplating the *T* word. Transplant or not, that was not in my control.

After six months of my new routine, I did not have a miraculous recovery; the lab results stated that it was indeed time to begin the evaluation process to be placed on the kidney transplant list. Once again, I couldn't get out of being human! We don't get to choose what life brings us, but we do get to choose what we do with it. My labs indicated that although my kidney function was down, my body was handling it well. I am thankful we have the luxury of being proactive about finding the right donor and preparing for kidney failure and transplant to avoid dialysis.

With all our unpredictable imperfection, illness prompts us to embrace our humanity and learn to get through our challenges instead of getting out of them. When you are at the mercy of your humanity, look back and think about what is in your control, and in a chronically resilient way, place your attention there.

Here are some things you can control:

- Living by your values (chapter 2)

- Making the most of your time (chapter 2)

- Listening the first time your body says it needs to rest (chapter 2)

- Finally doing what you've always wanted to (chapter 3)

- Learning relaxation techniques (chapter 4)

- Expressing your feelings (chapter 4)

- Turning away from worry (chapter 4)

- Keeping a peaceful home (chapter 5)

- Planning your meals and stocking the pantry (chapter 5)

- Preparing for hospital visits (chapter 5)

- Finding support (chapter 6)

- Being kind to those around you (chapter 6)

- Knowing when to bring in a professional coach or therapist (chapter 6)

- Educating yourself about your diagnosis (chapter 7)

- Finding a kick-butt medical team (chapter 7)

- Organizing your medical records (chapter 7)

- Bringing your thoughts back into the present moment (chapter 8)

- Taking your medications like your doctor thinks you are (chapter 9)

- Sticking to healthy standards: moving your body, keeping up with doctor appointments, practicing deep breathing, etc. (chapter 9)

- Measuring your accomplishments (chapter 9)

- Practicing self-forgiveness (chapter 9)

- Being grateful (chapter 10)

For your first journal exercise, make a list of things you can control. Start now, and add to the list as you continuing reading.

IN MY CONTROL

Start a list of all the things that are in your control. Add to it as you read or think of more.

Take back your life—take back responsibility for what is in your control. Owners take action; they lead, they provide motivation, and resolve. They assign meaning and make decisions. They control what they can and trust that they will have the strength and resources to move through the rest.

Is ownership tough? How about when you are tired, sick, and in pain? Yes, at times it is tough. There are times when all your strength is gone and you want to hand the reins over to someone or something else. You want to wallow; you want to cry; you want to get angry and stuff your face with pie. Ownership does not mean those feelings go away; it means you use them as a catalyst to change, to grow, and to investigate who you truly are. Not what the lab results say, not what the MRIs show, but who you are at your core.

I ask again, "why me?" I have an illness because I am human. It requires me to be patient and compassionate with myself. It challenges me to control what I can and accept what I can't. It helps me see what is important and let go of the trivial stuff. It shows me that I am much more than my body. It is my teacher, and I am here to learn.

A Conversation with Meredith Israel Thomas, Breast Cancer Warrior

Featured on CBS and NBC, Meredith Israel Thomas courageously shaved her head in front of millions of people prior to starting chemotherapy. She has raised more than $100,000 for cancer research and continues to advocate for early detection. Visit her at: *www.caringbridge.org/ visit/meredithisrael.*

"'You have some spots. They look suspicious.' That word [suspicious] to me, now, is the worst word you could ever imagine. Suspicious. More or less, they already know you have cancer."

The day after her thirty-sixth birthday, Meredith Israel Thomas learned that her diagnosis of stage 2 breast cancer was really stage 4. It had spread into her liver and bones. "He told me stage 4; he gave me less than a year. And that's when everything hit. To have a doctor give you less than a year to live, and Niomi [her daughter] was only eighteen months old. That night, everyone left the house, and I collapsed in my brother's arms, and I said, 'Why is it always me?'"

But Meredith stayed strong, thanks to her mantra, "Kick cancer's ass!"

That attitude has turned her one-year prognosis into a three-year-and-counting journey of treatments, trials, and living life. As Meredith says, "It's a stairwell to me. You take one step up, two steps back."

I learned about Meredith from *The Today Show*, where she took control and shaved her head in front of millions of people in preparation for chemotherapy treatments. She was going to fight cancer on her own terms. With a voice that conveys the strength of the warrior she is, she spoke with me about taking ownership.

Meredith was visiting her cancer treatment center for the first time, and she was not impressed with her doctor's demeanor. As she puts it, "She was just so forward, and ugh . . . just so harsh. Finally, I turned to the doctor after the next few appointments and I said, 'Listen. I'm a mother and I'm a person, and you need to have some relationship with me.' The doctor turned to me and said, 'I can't be your friend. I have to be your doctor.' I replied, 'Well, you have to talk to me nicer.'" In the end, speaking up for herself proved to be the beginning of a caring friendship with that same doctor.

Meredith attributes her strength and ability to take ownership in her fight against cancer to her earlier battle with postpartum depression. Due to a disorder from her childhood, Meredith was told she would be unable to have children. Getting pregnant with her daughter Niomi was a miracle. When postpartum depression "stole three months" from Meredith after Niomi's birth, she got pissed. "I would sit outside and scream at God that I had always wanted a child and now he's taking [this experience] away from me. So when this [cancer] happened, I just said 'no!'"

Meredith was determined not to lose. Still, she is realistic about the prognosis. As she puts it, "I am not one of those people who sugarcoats it, who says they're going to find a cure. They should have had a cure by now. I am very realistic. The cure is not coming in my time, but that doesn't mean I'm going to roll over like a lot of other patients do. There are patients who just lay down and are done and the cancer wins. It's crazy. I've now known two people who said, 'I'm not going to fight,' and in a week, they're dead." Meredith is determined, more than anyone

I have seen, to squeeze as much life as she can out of her time here.

When I asked her what was in her control, Meredith's first reaction—the reaction a lot of us have—was, "Nothing's really in my control. Physically, nothing's in my control." After a soft pause, though, she started to make a list of what *was* in her control. Meredith's cancer has spread to her bones, and early on she learned that a hug can crack a rib. The first thing on her list was being careful.

"I know where the cancer's located, and I'm careful. I'm careful with picking up Niomi, I'm careful with heavy packages. I'm in control of mentally staying strong for those around me. The only thing I'm in control of is continuing to live life, because you can walk around with the 'Woe is me, I'm a cancer patient' attitude, or you can take it and change your life like I did.

"What I've learned through all my friends is that you have to own it. When I shaved my head, there was no hiding from anybody now. It's fully on display: I'm bald. You can't hide it. I took control of that."

The highest priority on Meredith's list of responsibilities is staying strong for her daughter. She is fierce about caring for and shielding Niomi from the horrors of cancer. "For Niomi's sake, I need to be in control of how I act in front of her."

When it comes to controlling the progression of cancer, Meredith turns to her mind. "I have no control except for mentally telling you [the cancer] to get out of me. That 'I'm going to beat you,' and talking to it. When I feel a pain, it's like a ping. I sometimes picture the shotguns going right around that area. I think, 'OK, we're going to blast you.' Unfortunately, deep down, you have no control, but I do think that from all the survivors I've met, the stronger ones mentally seem to last longer because they're just not throwing in the towel.

"I've been very open with everybody; I know when I'm going to throw in the towel. There have been days when the medicine gets to be too much and I've said, 'Enough,' and I allow myself to cry that day. And then I pick up Niomi from school, and I kick myself back in gear. But I've been very clear with everybody, 'There will be no pain and suffering. I've already been through enough and [ask that you] don't extend my life because you guys need me.'

"I suffer every day. Every morning the first thing I think about is the cancer. I wake up and think, 'OK. I'm here, and I'm not sick today,' but it never goes away. So, I guess, I just own my life."

Meredith knows she can control what she does with each day here on earth, and that's when the bucket list started. "When I got diagnosed, this bucket list just formed in my head, and skydiving was the first thing I thought of doing. I e-mailed [a family friend and skydiver] and told him, and he said, 'Get up here!' My mom was with us, and we went skydiving. And it was my step to kicking it back, saying, 'I'm still here.' It was so exciting!"

Also on the list was getting a tattoo. The first tattoo she got before chemotherapy was "warrior" in Hebrew. The tattoo solidarity spread with her mom, cousins, aunt, dad, brother, and sister-in-law all getting them. She says getting a tattoo is "as addicting as everyone says." Since then, Meredith has added a second tattoo that says "unconditional love."

"To me, it is so powerful, because I look at Gary [Meredith's husband], and since Gary met me, between getting pregnant, postpartum depression, moving to New York, buying a house, breast cancer, all of this stuff, I would have run for my life if I were him, and he hasn't budged. That, to me, is just unconditional love."

When Meredith learned that hormone therapy hadn't worked and chemotherapy was the next step in her cancer treatment plan, she decided to lose her hair on her own terms. Through her contacts she got hooked up with *The Today Show*. "I really did not want to lose my hair, and I just said, 'I'm doing it,' [shaving my head on TV] and *a lot* of people disagreed with me. 'Wait 'til it falls out,' 'Wait 'til you lose a chunk.' I couldn't imagine seeing chunks of my hair falling out and shedding. I mean, everyone, including the wig place, said, 'You should be waiting.' Other patients told me I was stupid. I just said, 'I have to do it my way.' I called a couple of survivors . . . and it happened.

"I called my haircutter and said, 'So are you ready to shave it now?' and she said, 'No, but I'm going to do whatever you ask me to do.' We all gathered, and talked, and there were a lot of tears that day. I just wanted it over with. I got the tattoo, I shaved my head, I got a wig. I did it my way, and I still have no regrets. I didn't fully lose my hair in the end, so that was the joke. But I had bald spots, so I would have had to shave it because I wouldn't have wanted it to be like that."

> I'm not as dramatic as I always was. I just laugh at certain things now. We, as Americans, are just workaholics to an obnoxious level, but there is so much more. Now I can't sweat the small stuff.

Meredith says cancer has changed her outlook on life. "I'm not as dramatic as I always was. I was so dramatic. Everything was a drama. I think I changed after the postpartum depression, but I definitely changed after the cancer. I have no patience for dumb stuff anymore. I can't deal with drama now. The other thing I've learned is [about] work. I was always a workaholic, and I'll never forget, with one of my [publicity company] bands or opening up a restaurant, people would start yelling, and

I'd think 'What the fuck? We're not curing cancer here; it's opening a restaurant.' And now I definitely look at it like that. I just laugh at certain things now. I understand work. We, as Americans, are just workaholics to an obnoxious level, but there is so much more. Now I can't sweat the small stuff. I can't deal with drama like that. It's just ridiculous because there's so much more out there."

Meredith's motivation to retain her health is also her wakeup call. "Every morning I hear Niomi's footsteps running from her room to mine, and she pulls the blanket down and says, 'Good morning, Mommy!' I just start laughing. I mean, it cracks me up. When she says, 'I love you' and hugs me, I feel like Niomi's been through so much because of this. She's honestly why I fight. She deserves to have me around. There's nothing like a mommy. She loves her daddy, but there's nothing like a mommy. I use that as my strength, and that's why I've told them, 'No suffering!' I don't want her to ever see that side."

Meredith demonstrates the essence of ownership: living life. She has refused to let cancer take over. She remains resilient "just by living life regularly," and she fills her time doing normal things: going to movies, reading books, and, she confesses, "I'm still a TVaholic." Managing cancer along with running her own publicity company was not possible, so Meredith closed her company to focus on her health. However, she found it was important to have things to look forward to when she was feeling good. She is now volunteering at a children's foundation, where they understand her situation. "They know I might not show up some days, and they know other days I'm going to be rocking it." And rock it she does.

With exceptional courage and grace, Meredith has devoted her life to writing and advocating for cancer prevention, detection, and research so that one day her daughter will live in a world that has even more ownership over the fight with cancer.

HEALTH TIPS

- Recognize that challenges are part of the human journey.

- Take ownership of your body by accepting responsibility for your health.

- Focus on what is in your control.

- Take action on things that are in your control.

- Have compassion for yourself and the journey you are on.

CHAPTER 2

Identify and Live
Your Values

My uncle bought a special set of dolls for me when I was young, and I housed them in a delicate wooden box from my mom's childhood. On the top was a painted scene of pastel rolling hills surrounded by intricately carved Elizabethan leaves and vines. It latched with a tiny tarnished bronze clasp. Inside, six-inch hand sewn dolls were all squished together; legs were on heads, arms flailed about. The dolls portrayed all sorts of characters: a policeman, an Indian, a cowboy—my very own little set of Village People.

I only brought the dolls out occasionally, and never when another playmate was around. They were all mine. I took extra care to protect them from spills, and they never got to go on backyard camping trips like my Barbies did. I would spend hours imagining the dolls were in class led by the six-inch stuffed schoolteacher. Even though I was young, I understood the significance of having the dolls put in my care. No one needed to tell me they were special. I just knew, and I valued them.

How often do we extend the same level of care to our own lives? It is a rare thing to hold ourselves with the same gentle touch I used to hold my dolls. Learning how is part of living with illness.

Take Inventory

If you have ever worked retail, you have probably spent a late evening taking inventory. Armed with a pen, a list of products, and a scanner, you methodically count and recount product on the store shelves and in the stock room. Shirts–44, Socks–22, Pants–35, Dresses–18 . . . and so the night goes, until everything is accounted for.

Your life can be seen as a set of inventory shelves neatly stacked with boxes. Each box represents one hour of each day. Your personal inventory is the collection of activities you do with the hours in your day. If you work eight hours per day, Monday through Friday, then you have forty hours of work inventory in your week.

Some of the activities in your life hold a lot of meaning; others, not so much. Perhaps you do some things because you're too polite to say no, or you feel as if things won't get done unless you do them yourself. The hours in your day may seem like a repetitive jumble of events, but each hour is a representation of your value system. For example, Starbucks makes coffee. They spend an enormous amount of time making coffee. You may think their business is only about making coffee, but in Starbucks' culture, coffee is a metaphor. The first line of their mission statement is: "To inspire and nurture the human spirit—one person, one cup and one neighborhood at a time."[2] Your grande, half caf, extra hot, one-pump caramel soy latte is served up to inspire and nurture your spirit.

---

2 Starbucks' Mission Statement. *www.starbucks.com.*

Values are the freedom you'd burn your bra for, the justice that calls you to march, and the love that made you say yes when your beloved was down on one knee. They are the principles you regard with importance. Your actions are the ways you express your values. Do you see a disconnect between what you claim to value and how you spend the hours in your day? You may say you value health, but if you work eighty hours a week, eat junk food, and let cobwebs collect on the treadmill, it is likely you value something entirely different more than health. It is unusual to actually think about the greater meaning behind the ins and outs of our day. We simply work, grocery shop, cook, eat, clean—a lot of time is spent cleaning—and go through the other mundane tasks required to keep life moving forward. We have moments of inspiration and make grand promises to focus on spirituality by meditating or to value contribution by volunteering, but the moment someone needs us, we will drop our agenda and leave our promises unmet.

We allow ourselves to be driven by things other than the values we subscribe to. We let motives such as "avoiding pain" or "fitting in" determine our actions. Take inventory to see what values your actions support.

Your Current Inventory

To assess your inventory, first grab your journal (yes, really, get up and go get it), and think back over last week. How were you spending your time? What values do you think your actions represent? If you are geeky like me and love Excel, you may want to create a chart to detail out a typical day. For example:

DAY	TIME	ACTIVITY	VALUE(S)
Monday	7:00–8:00 A.M.	slept-in, showered, got dressed	comfort, cleanliness
	8:00–5:00 P.M.	worked	money, creativity, accomplishment
	5:00–8:00 P.M.	dinner, family time	family
	8:00–10:00 P.M.	watched TV	entertainment, rest

If you are a free spirit, cherry-pick the things you do most often and write down what your motivation for doing them is. In your journal, you should now have written out a number of activities and the values (or obligations) that they stand for.

What is in alignment? Where is there disconnect? And what needs to adjust? ("Yikes, I value learning, but I can't say that watching *Jerseylicious* supports that!") Your values and mix of inventory will be as unique as you are. Sunday dinner with your family could be about honoring the value of connection, or it could symbolize the creative process of trying a new recipe. This is the time to let the schoolgirl perfectionist stuff go. There are no right answers. Really. I mean it.

YOUR CURRENT INVENTORY

Write down how you spent your time last week. For each activity list the corresponding value it represents. Look for insights and disconnects.

Time to Reorganize

Illness gets stressful when your body requires more of your time and attention than can be squeezed into an already full life. It is easy to feel pulled between the life you used to live and the new reality you are facing. Like a store clearing out its summer polka dot swimsuits for fall sweaters and jackets, you too need to reorganize your inventory in the wake of chronic illness. Keeping the activities that represent what's important and ditching the rest will help you get serious about how you spend the hours in each day.

TED (Technology, Engineering and Design) is a global set of conferences which bring together the best smarty-pants of our time to present their innovative ideas. Since its start, TED has spawned a movement and evolved into the impressive website *www.ted.com.* I highly recommend checking out the talk by Stacey Kramer.[3] Stacey is a stunning, petite blonde who begins her presentation by describing a gift. An image of a bright teal box with a white ribbon smartly tied into a bow on top is projected on the screen behind her. For Kramer, the gift inside was a collection of values: love, spirituality, faith, trust, vitality, and relaxation. The bright teal box with the bow was a brain tumor. She recognized that out of the toughest challenge of her life came the opportunity to return to the basics of what is important.

Have you ever wished that one fantastical day in the future your life would be perfect? You would be rich, healthy, dangerously attractive, wildly in love, and happy all the time. You are not quite sure how that is all going

---

3 Stacey Kramer, "The Best Gift I Ever Survived." Video (February, 2010). *www.ted.com.*

to come about, but someday you'll see what's at the end of the rainbow. This wish is quicksand. It keeps you waiting passively for your day in the sun, only to realize life's the same each evening as you get into bed. It prevents you from seeing that today is the only day you've got to make a difference in your life. If you put off being the woman you truly want to be, you will never give yourself the opportunity to do just that.

After you looked at your current inventory, were you shocked by how you spend your time and what that time represents? This is your chance to restock your inventory shelves, but in order to do so, you need to identify the values you want to live by going forward. Knowing what you stand for determines which activities make it into your day.

Ask the Big Questions

There are three big questions that will help you determine your values. Picture it: you're on Oprah's couch, she leans in, takes a long pause, and asks you:

What is important to you? What activities, people, interactions, and projects give you the most joy and satisfaction? What makes you feel fully alive? What makes time pass quickly? What would you choose to do with your free time? What do you feel fully committed to? What can you not live without?

What do you want to be remembered for? What will your legacy be? What sort of parent, child, spouse do you want to be? What do you want your work to stand for? What do you want others to receive from your work? How do you want others to feel after they interact with you?

What lessons are important for you to learn during your lifetime? How do you want to improve? What do you need to learn about relating to yourself? To others? What do you need to learn about trust? About love? What areas of personal growth are essential for you to explore?

Once you've answered these three big questions in your journal, take some time to review your answers. The themes, ideas, and hopes that you brought up in your answers are bright fluorescent arrows that point to what you value. Get more specific by expressing each value in a word or two. For instance, if painting watercolor pictures is what you would choose to do with your free time, the value would be creativity. Aim for five to ten values total; these will be the key values you will focus on. If you need some help putting your values into words, see Appendix A. I've listed a bunch there. Next, rank your values in order of priority, starting with the most important. This makes it obvious what you need to give the most time and energy to in your life.

IDENTIFY YOUR VALUES

Answer these three questions:

1. What's important to you?

2. What do you want to be remembered for?

3. What lessons are important for you to learn during your lifetime?

From your answers, list your top ten values in order of priority.

When I answered the question "What is important to you?" I was reminded of a drive Phillip and I took one late November. We had a free afternoon and decided to go to Lake Tahoe, a two-hour drive from our home. Forty-five minutes into our road trip, the trees stretched ten feet closer to the sun, the air cleared, and the forest sewed together as our car climbed into the Sierra Nevada Mountains. I immediately felt giddy. Every tree, stream, and boulder around me was electric. You have got to see the Sierras in the fall. The colors glide across the mountainside in a sunset of leaves. It was take-your-breath-away beautiful. I forget how important nature is to me until I am surrounded by it. It brings me . . . So. Much. Joy. A Nordstrom shopping spree will never give me more satisfaction than a ponderosa pine tree can.

The mountains were a big part of my childhood. All of our family vacations were at 10,000 feet with a few tents and a stream nearby. Early on, I learned to love the crisp air and serendipity of nature's details. That November day, I realized how much I valued being in nature. I knew that it was healing for me, and that I would need to mold my life around it more. Nature needed an inventory shelf all to itself.

Identifying your values helps you become deliberate about the actions you take. It gives you a measure to help you make decisions, pursue projects, and fill up your free time. When you know your values, you can put your schedule up against them and incessantly ask yourself, "Does this support my values?"

Value Yourself First

In her article "Top 5 Regrets of the Dying," Bronnie Ware, a palliative care nurse, writes that the most common regret she heard from patients was that they wanted to live life true to their own desires, not to the expectations of others.[4]

The initial inventory you took of your life may reflect many hours devoted to picking up socks, grocery shopping, organizing the bake sale, taking on an extra project at work, balancing budgets, and cooking dinner. Have you given yourself permission to take a break and heal? This was a lesson I had to remind myself of.

When I was little, my mom taught me about prioritizing myself. Anytime I was sick, getting well was number one. I never went to school with so much as a cough, even though I feared I would fall behind. Recovering my health became my mom's top priority, as it would for any mother. We saw specialists, tried new diets, put lifts in my shoes, went to faith healers, saw chiropractors, bought humidifiers, and did just about anything that had to do with going from sick to well. I saw firsthand what making health a priority looked like. However, right as I entered high school, I started to choose my own priorities, and they shifted to look more like obligations.

I was studious, and I put being a good student above my health. I started to get frequent kidney infections when I was sixteen, and I would hide my symptoms from my parents so that I could attend class, all cold sweat and nauseated. After school, I would drive to cheerleading practice with the car heater on full blast until my hands seared on the steering wheel to help with the chills. Even though my body was screaming for me to take a break, to see the doctor, to lie down, I pushed myself past my limits with little regard for how I felt. In fact, I misguidedly thought that I was being strong and

---

4 Bronnie Ware, "Top 5 Regrets of the Dying: A Palliative Care Nurse Shares What She Learned While Caring for Her Patients," *More* (2012, February). *www.more.com.*

courageous to continue on with life pretending that my body wasn't sick.

The height of my denial occurred when I was seventeen and had my first boyfriend. I thought that in order to be liked, I had to be an easy-breezy, make-no-demands sort of girl—one who didn't spoil plans by getting sick. On a sunny June morning, the plan was to go to SeaWorld. I also had a kidney infection. I spent the morning with chills and a fever in a searing hot shower, preparing to be on my feet all day as I walked to see the penguins and Shamu with my boyfriend and his family. I was too nauseated to eat breakfast, and by the time we arrived at the park I was starving. During lunch the only thing that sounded remotely appetizing was a bowl of strawberries, which, in retrospect, was not the smartest choice. As we got up from the lunch table, I had the undeniable queasy drool that comes just before you lose it. I headed straight for the bathroom. I didn't make it. My white Keds showed the strawberry-red evidence of just how sick I was. But did that stop me? No. It should have, but it didn't. I cleaned up and rejoined the family to fulfill my girlfriend duties. I could not admit that I needed to lie down. I could not admit that I wasn't superhuman. I refused to make myself my number one priority that day. After a few more attractions, and almost puking again during the sea lion show, my boyfriend insisted he take me home. By trying to make it through the day while being sick, I wasn't there for anyone.

When we insist that illness not impact our lives, we are shortchanging ourselves and everyone around us. Everything gets done half-assed. You are not present for

> You are not present for your family, your work, or anyone when you push past your limits for the sake of trying to keep things normal when they are decidedly not normal.

your family, your work, or anyone when you push past your limits for the sake of trying to keep things normal when they are decidedly not normal.

In the years following my SeaWorld incident, I have learned to be sick when I am nauseated, in pain, and feverish. I have learned to ask for what I need and make myself the priority my mom showed me I am.

Part of the reason we try to be all things to all people is our culture. Have you ever sat through a business meeting while someone is sniffling and sneezing and exposing everyone else to their cold? In that moment they are valuing achievement, money, or appearances above their health and the health of everyone else in the room. Have you ever made any of the following assumptions?

- I won't be respected if I take time off.

- Things will fall apart at home.

- It will look like a bomb went off in the house if I don't clean it.

- I'm not worth much if I'm sick.

- They can't do it without me.

- The project is more important than I am.

- This has to get done today.

- I will rest tomorrow.

- I can't ask for help.

- No one has time to help me.

- I can't miss this.

- My kids, husband, job, and everything else come first.

- I don't have time to be sick.

We yearn for the approval of others, and we mistakenly believe that in order to get it we have to put ourselves last. Women willingly sacrifice their health to service the desire for external achievement. Would you ever tell a friend that she's "not worth much" if she's sick?

Getting sick is your body's way of telling you that things need to change. Please give yourself permission to listen to your body. Give yourself permission to need healing. Allow your health to become a priority. You cannot build a life around your values unless you decide that *you* are also of value.

Living by your values means that you are not going to let circumstances, obstacles, or fears determine how your life is lived. Other people's demands and external obligations will need to come under the scrutiny of your values system. Remember to ask yourself, "Does this support my values?" If you don't believe that you are of value, you will allow other people to spend your time and energy on what they value.

This isn't to say that you can never help your kids with their homework, cook dinner for your husband, or work late. It is about shifting your perspective to see what is behind your actions. Helping the kids with their homework may speak to the values of family and education. Cooking dinner can be about creativity, health, and love. Working late can represent diligence, loyalty, or commitment. When you face a decision about how to spend your time, check in with yourself to see if it falls in line with your current state of health and what you value most.

> Living by your values means that you are not going to let circumstances, obstacles, or fears determine how your life is lived.

My mom taught me that I was born with a high-maintenance body, one that needs extra care and attention, and calls me to become a priority in my life. Your body is just the same.

Live Your Values

Go back to your journal and look over what you listed as your top five or ten values. It is time to reorganize your inventory to find more shelf space for these.

Clean Out

Before you place your values up on your shelves, you need to purge what you don't need anymore, the things that take your time, your energy, and your sanity without adding to your life. In your journal, make a list of everything that goes out to the curb for trash day. Here are a few of my favorites:

- Wasting hours reading horrific side effects and worst-case scenarios of your illness on the Internet. (We'll talk more about this in chapter 7.)

- Getting in a tizzy over small things.

- Attempting to control other people's problems.

- Stressing about what your health might be like tomorrow, a week from now, or next year.

- Watching mindless TV. (The shows you feel guilty for watching and the ones that make you scared to be home alone.)

- Buying into drama in all its glorious forms.

- Putting things on your to-do list that will never get done.

- Hanging around unsupportive people.

- Sorrow-drowning in junk food.

- Making excuses.

- Getting buried in relentless e-mail newsletters and spam.

- Feeling guilty about being in groups you never attend.

Go at your life with a weed whacker, relentlessly trimming away the stuff that isn't important. If you feel drained after an activity, it has to go. You need all of your energy pointed toward maintaining your health and enjoying life.

CLEAN OUT

List all of the things you will eliminate from your life to make room for your newly identified values.

Consider Big Changes

After you've filled a few black bags with old inventory, go a bit deeper. There may be things that you do now out of duty or obligation that don't fulfill you and may negatively impact your health. These are the tougher choices. I say tougher because letting them go may involve facing some heart-pounding moments. For instance, if you have a job that is taking more than it's giving you, you may need to take time off, rearrange your work schedule, or find a new position altogether. This probably means adjusting your household budget, moving, learning new skills, or putting that shiny new car on hold—or a combination of these. We'll talk more about finances in chapter 6.

Leaving corporate America was terrifying. My job in finance was secure, and I was good at it, but I wanted to take my career in a more creative direction that allowed me time and space to focus on my health. My favorite part of school, and later, my work, had always been giving presentations, and I dreamt of building a career around speaking and writing. I baby-stepped my way into my own business by starting the website, *www.creativeaffirmations.com*, on the side. When I finally made the transition to being self-employed, my blood pressure dropped and I was able to cut my blood pressure medication dose in half.

Letting go of big things that push on your sense of security takes extra planning and creative thinking, but these changes can have a massive payoff. What is the sense in working tirelessly for a huge house if you won't have the health to enjoy it? If you feel that a change of this magnitude is in order, it's time for a family meeting to discuss options for how you can adjust your lifestyle to accommodate your new path. We will discuss setting goals more in the next chapter.

CONSIDER BIG CHANGES

Jot down a few ideas in your journal of what making "big changes" might involve. This is just brainstorming at this point—you'll have time to really consider these ideas later on.

Delegate

Don't stress yourself out; you don't have to do it all. Decide what someone else can do. Your health depends on letting people help you. In your journal, make a list of all the things you take care of. Next, divide the list into things that require your expertise and things other people can do. What can your husband, children, and relatives do? How about friends or members of your community? What professional services could you hire?

Look over your list of items to delegate, and decide a schedule of who will do what and when.

Consider hiring a cleaning service. Seriously. It is estimated that a woman spends the bulk of her free time cleaning, and one-third of women feel uncomfortable delegating cleaning tasks to their spouses.[5] We need to get over it. It is OK if the dishes go undone for a night and the laundry turns into a mini-Everest. You can always shut the closet door. The bulk of the time you spend cleaning could be spent on getting better, especially if you also work full time. If finances are tight, look into a volunteer cleaning service. Cleaning for a Reason (*www.cleaningforareason .org*) is a nonprofit organization that partners with local cleaning companies to provide services to women healing from cancer. Even hiring a professional to come in for a one-time deep cleaning can make a big difference.

There are all sorts of other things besides cleaning that you can delegate to carve out more time to focus on your values. Here are a few ideas to get you started:

- Grocery shopping

- Taking out the trash

- Yard work

- Managing finances

- Getting and sorting the mail

- Cooking

- Carpooling with other parents to get the kids here and there

- Dealing with the insurance company

---

5 Julia Edelstein, "What Women Can't Let Go." *Real Simple* (April, 2012). *www.realsimple.com.*

By letting go, making big changes, and delegating, you have cleared a few shelves to spend time on your personal values. Now, how to fill that up?

Schedule Sacred Time

Identify some time each day that is just for you to do with as you please. It is helpful to pick a consistent time each day so that you and your family get in the habit of knowing that 8:00 to 9:00 each evening (or whatever time you choose) is just for you. You can meditate, take a hot bath, read, scrapbook, work out, or whatever else eases stress and gives you energy. View this time as being just as important as your other obligations. If you had to be at work each day by 8:00 A.M., I am sure there is little that would keep you from being there. Look at your sacred time the same way. It is as vital to your wellness as your medications and doctor visits.

Be Idealistic

Think about what an ideal day would look like if the bulk of your time were spent honoring your top three to five values. If you work, you may want to complete this exercise for a weekday and a weekend day. On a fresh page of your journal, detail all of the activities you would put into that day, from your first cup of coffee to turning out the light. It doesn't matter if it isn't realistic—in fact, if it's not, that's even better. This is a day only for you, where everyone around you is obliged to do what you want to do.

> **MY IDEAL DAY**
>
> Detail what a day dedicated 100 percent to you and your favorite things would consist of from morning until evening. You may choose to do this exercise for a weekday and a weekend day. List ways you can incorporate elements of your ideal day into your every day.

Once you have written the ending to your ideal day, preferably on silk sheets, under a plump down comforter, and sleeping peacefully, ask "how can I incorporate elements of my ideal day into every day?" If, like me, nature is your sanctuary and your ideal day includes a walk in the woods, this may not be practical as an everyday occurrence. But you could still have your morning coffee outside, eat lunch under a tree in the park, or add an orchid to your office. Consider the meaning behind the activities in your ideal day and find practical ways to apply them.

Revamp your daily schedule to allow yourself to focus on your values. Stock your shelves with the activities, interactions, and people that help you live as true to yourself as possible. Keep in mind that choosing to live your values is not a onetime decision. It is a choice you will have to make again and again. Continually check in with yourself to see if you are choosing love, choosing peace, choosing contribution, and choosing to live what is important to you.

Illness is your license to be as deliberate and thoughtful with your time as you want to. Live as you would live at the end of your life right now, today. That is the gift.

> Choosing to live your values is not a onetime decision. It is a choice you will make again and again.

A Conversation with Sarah Ramey, Singer and Songwriter Living with an Indeterminate Illness

Writer, singer, and songwriter Sarah Ramey has lived with an autoimmune-like illness for the past ten years. Her first album, *Quiet at the Kitchen Door*, is available at: *wolflarsenmusic.com*.

Ten years ago, Sarah Ramey went into the operating room to have a procedure done which promised to halt frequent urinary tract infections. But the surgery caused chronic pain and a brush with septic shock that "unleashed this other, bigger disease that I describe as a constellation of indeterminate autoimmune-like problems. It is quite a lot like rheumatoid arthritis, lupus, and a little bit like Lyme disease. It's not an autoimmune disease. It's this huge illness that has so many symptoms but at the same time no diagnosis."

The lack of a diagnosis has been one of the biggest challenges for Sarah. She says "when there's no name, it's very hard to just say that I've got 'randomness terribleolis,' and everyone would reply, 'oh, no!' Instead, I say, 'yeah, I'm really sick,' and people reply, 'well, you don't look sick; you look great!'"

With very real fatigue, pain, and inflammation, Sarah revamped her life. "I had to quit my job. I was working as a writer for Obama during his first presidential campaign. It was a dream job. When I did that, I was home for a while. It was such a blow to not be able to keep going, and to not get any answers in Western medicine, that I moved to San Francisco. I started seeing an acupuncturist two times a week and a homeopath and I started doing yoga. I went all for it with green juice—the whole thing. It helped a lot, and I definitely improved. I went from waif-like to way more vital, but I was still going through an enormous amount of pain and no bowel function, this 'over-problem' of feeling sick all of the time."

With such drastic lifestyle changes, it is clear that Sarah had centered her life on the things that are most important to her. I asked her, "How do you practice valuing yourself?" She says, "That has definitely been something that I've done in a couple of different ways. One is a really well defined routine of self-care and prioritizing, even though my priority isn't everybody else's. For a while, I would not do that; I would pretend like I was OK. I would do everything that everyone else was doing, and I have scaled way back from doing that, which has been very helpful. I also honor myself because you get to this point where you realize, OK, I am a little bit different, and I need to take care of myself. I meditate, and my diet is very tailored to what works for me. I exercise and I try to be in nature.

"Another really good part has been my business. I'm a writer and a musician. So if I'm going to have this really, really debilitating illness, I'm definitely going to write the book that I want to write, and I'm definitely going to write music because if it's going to be like this, then it's up to me to infuse this life with as much positive and meaningful stuff as I can so that some of it feels good.

"Permission is a big part of it. That's a scary step for a lot of people to take. [People think,] 'Oh, I'm allowed to do what I really feel called to do?' It feels bad or it feels selfish, and then you start doing it, and it's not. It's just what you do."

Sarah had a history of singing in other people's bands or choir. Once she moved to San Francisco, she says she was "kind of improving, but not at the rate I thought I was going to. I was really a shut-in." Someone suggested she look into the open mike nights at the Hotel Utah, a great local club, and "one night something snapped. I thought, I've got to get out of here. I can't take this anymore. I threw my guitar in the car and I went down there and played a Leonard Cohen medley. I met all these people. It was great!"

That night Sarah invented her stage name: Wolf Larsen. She thought "This is my chance. Nobody knows me here. I think I'm going to go with Wolf Larsen [after her grandfather]. It was the most awkward but empowering thing I think I have ever done, to step outside myself and create this. I forget my illness and just enjoy getting to play." Singing at the Hotel Utah became a weekly outlet for Sarah. Eventually she joined a songwriting challenge. "I wrote my first song, and then I kept going for another year, got to practice, and started playing gigs. I started to become a lot more serious about it, and then last year we recorded."

It is obvious that music is instrumental for Sarah to honor her health; it is a gift in her life. I asked her about her gift, and after a contemplative pause, she replied,

"It's definitely an outlet for expression, which is sort of trite, but I think it's very true. [My record] is not an upbeat record. It's very much a place to put a lot of what has been really difficult and also very difficult to express. It has definitely been a place to get that out in a way that feels like transmuting it into something else. It's something to do with all of that energy instead of just holding on to it." Her performances allow her to let go of her "darker energy" again and again so that she doesn't "have to hold on to it anymore." Sarah's voice is intentional, melodic, and filled with honesty as she sings "No was her name. / No was the lion that no one could tame." Her music is the vessel that she pours herself into. Each note carries the pain and insight of a long and winding journey.

Sarah considers "feeling alive" to be the most important aspect of being on this earth. "Even if that means feeling in pain or feeling sick, but just being present to it. Being alive. There's always something right next to you that's a way to expand outward to feel more alive and to feel lucky that you're alive, even if it sucks at that point." That feeling of aliveness comes from a few different places for Sarah: "feeling of service, feeling really, truly connected to other people (and) important people in my life." She also takes extra care to make sure that the food she eats makes her "feel alive, and not the opposite."

With a routine that involves a specific diet and a variety of healing practices, how does Sarah make time for those activities that help her feel alive? For her it starts with being proactive. "It's not something that just happens. That's something that I have definitely learned, designing your life so that it is about the larger things. I have a life [where] I'm not working eighteen hours a day writing for somebody else. I'm writing for myself, and I've structured it so that I have the time to take care of myself. I do think that's a process. My illness is, honestly, overwhelming in so many ways. It's important to guard that time." She sees scheduling and practicality as paramount to keeping her health a priority. Over the years of coping with her illness, she has learned how her energy works, and she has learned to work around that. "It's been very helpful to me to honor what's particular to me."

One of the most important realizations Sarah has had on her journey is that there is "no diet plan or health guru that knows the answer. There are a lot of really good ideas out there, but everybody is so individual. It's important to give yourself permission to honor that, to really listen to what does work and what doesn't and scheduling that. Be serious about it."

This has extended to a lesson in self-compassion. She reflects, "It's OK that I don't find a miraculous cure every day that I wake up; [I am] really getting better at living in the now and living in a way that feels good."

Getting into the world of alternative healing introduced Sarah to the metaphysical philosophy that the answer to why a person is sick lies in her emotional core. She did lots of self-examination to search for the chink in her emotions. She remembers, "That, in and of itself was a very painful emotional journey of being constantly told, 'there's got to be something terrible in there [in her psyche] that's making you sick.' I really do believe that the body holds emotions as a real, physical component to it. I also think it's very helpful to not look at it as something wrong with you that you're trying to fix. Something bad happened, and yeah, maybe because I've had this issue and that issue now it's compounded. But here we are. It's certainly not serving the higher goal to think about it all the time, to explore it all the time. For me it's way more empowering to take action and do something in the world instead of sitting around and thinking about why. You can't know why."

The action she took was to sing in a way that brings tears to your eyes.

HEALTH TIPS

- Make yourself, and your health, a top priority.

- Let go of the things that needlessly spend your time and energy.

- Consider making big changes.

- Revamp your daily schedule to integrate your values.

- Constantly choose to live by your values.

CHAPTER 3

Set Attainable, Inspiring Goals

I wanted to be on show cheer in high school. You've seen the ESPN competitions—teams of male and female cheerleaders perform all sorts of lifts, pyramids, flips, and stunts in unison to a crowd that is going wild. As an added bonus, my high school show cheer team had lots of cute muscular guys who could lift you right over their head.

My congenital dislocated hip and scoliosis never stopped me from dancing. Ballet as a kindergartener was first, followed by tap and jazz. I stand a bit lopsided, but I danced anyway. When it came time for show cheer tryouts, I got right up there on the hands of two of my male schoolmates as they hoisted my feet up toward their chest. The team coach came over to check out my mid-air frozen jumping jack and commented, "You're leaning." I tried to straighten out, but to no avail. The guys' hands were even, it was my hip and spine that were askew. Later during the tryouts, girls backflipped and handspringed across the floor, something I could decidedly not attempt. It wasn't a surprise when I didn't make the team.

While my initial goal was show cheer, my body was simply not going there. I had to readjust. I set my sights on a new goal: cheerleading. No flipping required at my school. Their tryouts came next, and this time I made the team. No death-defying stunts and no boys, but an amazing group of girls and the opportunity to dance and cheer on my school. Participating in cheerleading kept my back muscles loose and gave me a great extracurricular outlet that helped to maintain my health. Goal adjusted.

I know my example above is a little, well, high school. Yet, at fifteen, it seemed the rotation of the earth hinged on my ability to make show cheer. Overly dramatic, yes. Definitely not as dramatic as some of the goals that will need to be rerouted when you are facing cancer, diabetes, MS, or any other chronic illness. Big, small, or somewhere in between, goals will need to shift when you get sick. Illness is the obnoxious orange detour arrow that causes you to modify your route. Even though there may be limitations, you still have the ability to change course and adjust your goals to fit your body and energy level.

> Illness is the obnoxious orange detour arrow that causes you to modify your route. Even though there may be limitations, you still have the ability to change course and adjust your goals to fit your body and energy level.

Without goals, even the itty-bitty ones, we wouldn't accomplish anything in life. Your entire day is one string of goal accomplishment: get out of bed, brush off the morning breath, eat breakfast, drive to the office, and on and on until the goal is to turn the lights out at night. You are an expert at creating and accomplishing goals. The purpose of this chapter is to put a few brain cells behind where you want to aim your life to ensure that you get to stand at the top of the pyramid if that is where you want to be, illness or not.

The Wheel of Health

If you have ever seen a life coach, you've probably filled out a Wheel of Life. It is an assessment where you determine how fulfilled you are in each area of your life. Coaches typically use eight areas of life, and the wheel looks something like this:

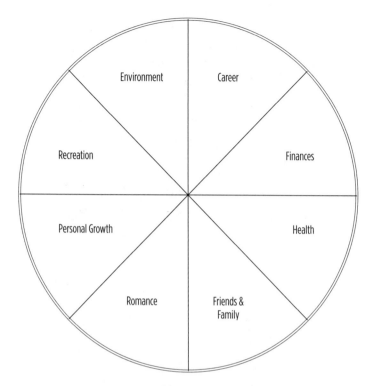

The philosophy behind the chart is that your whole life is the circle. To have the ultimate balanced and fulfilling life, you have to optimize each area within. That is a lot to take on! I get the intention behind this exercise, but did anyone tell these coaches that there are only twenty-four hours in each day?

A more accurate, and achievable, model is to look at the chart above in comparison to the whole span of your lifetime. As you grow, you move through phases. For example: When you are young, there is a larger focus on career than when you are retired. At the start of a relationship, romance is a big piece of a woman's life. While raising young kids, the bulk of the wheel is devoted to family.

Years ago, Phillip and I ventured back to an alumni reunion for our university and met a man who had graduated from our alma mater in the fifties. He told us that his fiftieth college reunion was the best because he now had the time to reconnect with all of his old friends. You don't have to focus on all eight areas of life all at once. That's not real life. For those of us who are ill, health needs a bigger piece of the pie, but it doesn't have to take over. "Illness meringue" doesn't taste very good.

Do you spend a lot of time thinking about why you got sick? How to get well? And if the itch behind your left knee is a new symptom? Your health can play freeze tag with every other area of your life, resulting in a wheel that looks like this:

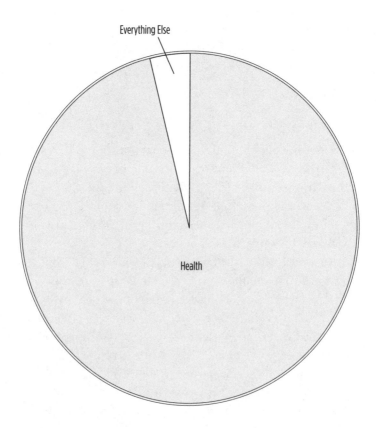

You don't need to add back in all seven other areas of life, but you do need to add some. Like Goldilocks, you're searching for "just right." If you are still breathing, you have life left to live, a life that is about much more than your health. You have people who you care about and who care about you. You have the capacity to contribute, even if the nature of your contribution needs to change. A diagnosis does not mean that things are over. It simply means that a detour arrow is in your path.

Do I Really Have to Set Goals?

Are you thinking, "Seriously? You're going to tell me I need to have goals when I don't feel well?" You bet I am.

Getting a diagnosis is a loss. You are losing the body and the life you knew. That loss can wipe clear a future that once seemed full and planned to a tee. This is scary, there's no denying it. However, leaving your future blank allows a diagnosis to crowd out your life.

While you may have lost the life you had yesterday, you can create something new. Goals are a commitment to the rest of your life. They will give you something to fight for. Your dreams are what give you the resolve to find your way past that glaringly persistent detour arrow.

In chapter 1, I suggested you stop pushing against and accept your diagnosis. Without goals, acceptance has the tendency to become indifference. Goals help you think, "I have an obstacle in my life, and I will do what I need to do to deal with it," instead of "I have this obstacle in my life, so why bother?"

Of the thirteen popular New Year's resolutions listed on *USA.gov*, three have to do with getting healthy: lose weight, eat healthy, and get fit. Let's be honest. "Get healthy" is not a very motivating goal. It will not get you to drink something dark green and power walk each day. "Get healthy" is a goal that will get you to procrastinate. The shove you need comes from what being healthier can give you. The extra energy that you have to play with your kids, the mobility to visit a new city, the lung capacity to take the hike, the sexiness that has your husband grabbing you from behind is what will increase your follow through.

"Love" is an atrociously inadequate word to describe the depth of emotion I have for Phillip. I am connected and devoted to my husband in fierce ways. I have a goal of sitting on the porch with him, holding hands, grandkids playing in the yard when we are in our seventies. I am going to do what needs to be done to live the day I've got in my mind. Eat green stuff, replace my organs, work out, whatever. When you replace "get healthy" with spend an extra moment with my daughter, or visit Machu Picchu, or start my own bakery, then you've got ammunition. Knowing *why* you want to maintain your health is essential to following your care plans. So, yes, you do have to set goals.

> The extra energy that you have to play with your kids, the mobility to visit a new city, the lung capacity to take the hike, the sexiness that has your husband grabbing you from behind is what will increase your follow through.

Goal setting is going to look different from when you were in the prime of health, if you ever were. You will have to be more creative with your goals, or at a minimum, give up being a stick-in-the-mud about how you approach them. I used to set elaborate goals with one- and five-year timelines. My inner perfectionist would detail everything out for each area of my life. Then I would put my goals in a drawer and never take action toward them. A few years later, I would do the whole exercise over again only to stack this new list on top of the last one.

The word of the day, every day, with illness is *simplify*. Setting lengthy goals you'll never accomplish is too much for anyone. You don't need to attempt to detail out each day of the next five years; you already know that life can easily throw a wrench in your plans. Instead create a list of ways that you'd like to experience and express your unique set of values (gathered in chapter 2)—no pressure, no timeline, just imagination.

> The word of the day, every day, with illness is *simplify*.

This will give you something to work toward when you feel up to it and give you the flexibility to put your goals aside and rest when necessary.

Illness opens up your life to a number of external influences and demands; it can feel as if your life is no longer your own. A few well-placed goals can reclaim your sense of self and direction. They help you retain independence.

Like a sticky peanut butter and jelly, it is easy to sandwich our ability to be productive with our health status. When your health is not 100 percent, you can feel defeated in your finances, career, relationships, and personal growth as well. Your body is not who you are. It is only one aspect of who you are. The goal setting process is the exploration of the whole of you, a decision about how you want to express yourself out in the world. The trick is to continue having dreams that point toward the future, but in a way that allows for extra personal care and compassion.

Four-Step Goal Setting

A few years ago, my first published magazine article arrived in the mail. It was in *RenaLife* magazine, a beautiful spread with glossy pictures and Danea Horn on the byline. Super-duper squealing exciting! On that same day, I was packing up our house for one of our many big moves. I was up in the bedroom throwing the contents of my nightstand into a box when an index card fell out. It said "Become a published author." The timing was uncanny. I barely remembered writing the index card. It must have been incubating in my nightstand for years.

When it was time to go through transplant testing, one of my first thoughts was, "wait, I have so many plans." There were all those other goals stacked in the other drawers that I had wanted to do for years but for some reason kept putting off, and now it felt like time was creeping up on me. Stop waiting for the right time, the right body, the right companion, the right finances, the right education. Whatever it is, today is the day to take a step toward it.

FOUR-STEP GOAL SETTING

1. Envision. Brainstorm all the goals you find intriguing.

2. Edit to five. Choose the five goals that are most inspiring and also attainable.

3. Check against values. Do your goals match up with your values identified in chapter 2?

4. Identify small actions. What steps can you take today or tomorrow that move you toward your goals?

My goal setting process is simple because I have found that the simpler your goals are, the easier they are to keep in a mind that is also keeping up with a diagnosis. No fancy-pants timelines or ten-point checklists. But don't limit yourself—you can state your goals in whichever way you want and get as original as you need to.

Step 1: Envision

Grab a cup of something warm and your journal, a few magazines, or your laptop and bolt your judgments away in a closet. Jot down as many things as you can think of that you want to do. Small things, big things, everything. Magazines and the Internet are helpful for generating ideas about things you didn't even know you wanted. Write and write and write until your hand cramps up. This is especially fun to do with a friend. You will feed off each other's ideas and steal a few for yourself. The only question you're answering right now is "What do I want?" That's it. Don't worry about having your goals be specific, positive, or in the present tense. Write them as you would talk to yourself.

Start with the future as a clean canvas and begin to mentally paint in what you want. This is not the time to list all of the reasons why you can't have what you want, just write them down. Start without expectations about what tomorrow *should* look like, and a different future than you are used to will emerge. Things that once seemed important in society's eyes (income, clothing, house, number of Facebook followers) may seem less so now. Particularly since you've done the work to identify your values, your goals will shift accordingly.

As you daydream, you may even come up with some interesting ways to express yourself. I once found myself in a rut and knew that I needed to shake things up. I wanted to get out of my comfort zone, so the goal I created was to try one new thing each week. That summer I visited an alpaca farm, tried tango and salsa dancing, took an improv class, and took mini me-time vacations. It was totally exhilarating!

> Start without expectations about what tomorrow *should* look like, and a different future than you are used to will emerge.

We tend to think in vanilla terms when the topic of goals comes up—house, car, relationship, or level of income—but no one has ever said that you can't have a goal to . . .

- Go away one weekend every few months.

- Have a weekly date night.

- Try a new recipe each week.

- Take a class: photography, cooking, painting, sewing, sculpture, etc.

- Try a new kind of dance. (Belly dancing, anyone?)

- Learn karate.

- Start a blog.

- Go on a meditation retreat.

- Host a dinner party each month.

- Meet one new person each week.

- Learn about your ancestry.

- Start a book club.

- Learn a new language.

- Try a new type of food.

- Write your life story.

- Donate time or money to a cherished organization.

- Learn to scuba dive.

The ideas can be endless. Check out your friends' Facebook or Pinterest accounts for additional inspiration.

Now that you have pages and pages of things you'd like to experience, it is time to do some editing.

Step 2: Edit to Five

The first swipe to take past your list is to delete any goals that are not your own. Even though you just wrote them down, some of your goals may be holdovers from what you think your spouse, parents, boss, society, or even doctors want you to do. If you set goals that are not what you really want, you won't give a darn to work toward them. Move through your list and ask, "Whose goal is this?" If the answer is anything but "all mine," cross it out.

The old adage that "you can do anything you put your mind to" is reaching. Filter by what is reasonable and attainable. Not that people don't accomplish astounding things every day, but having a goal that will push you further than you're willing to go can be frustrating, if not downright dangerous.

I spent a semester studying in Salzburg, Austria, and on a blue-sky Saturday afternoon, the student group I was part of decided to go hiking. I love to hike, but this wasn't a hike; it was a thigh-burning, torturous climb straight up the side of a mountain. I was embarrassed as eighty-year-old Austrian natives jogged up the trail past me who was paused, propped up against the handrail and gasping for air. A quarter of the way into the hike, and after numerous people asked me if I was OK, I realized that my lungs could not meet my goal. It was defeating to turn back and walk up the road to take the lift to the top where I met the victorious hikers. I had to be honest with myself about what my body could handle.

If you have a few goals that you feel really passionate about and think your body will throw a tantrum if you try them, before you cross them out, see if there is a compromise you could reach. My goal on the hike was to make it to the top of the mountain, which I did, even though I had to be carried up in a cable car. You may have the energy and ability to meet the challenges you set out for yourself if you are willing to be patient and reach your goal differently.

Now that your list is edited to reflect the goals that are yours and that are attainable for your level of health, the last thing to do is to pick five that you will put your focus on now. The goals that I have accomplished in my life were the ones that didn't have to fight for space on the bus. Your health takes a lot of your time and focus; it is important to keep room for that in your life. Once you have reached your first few goals, you can add in the next set of favorites from your list.

Step 3: Check Against Values

In the last chapter, we spent some time discovering what values you hold near and dear. Your goals are how you demonstrate your values in the world. For instance, the goal of a trip to Europe is a way to express adventure, discovery, relaxation—and if you go with someone you love, romance. Life becomes more fulfilling not when we are focused on maximizing every area of our lives, but when we are living life through our values.

Your top five goals need a values check. Turn back a few pages in your journal to where you listed your top ten values. For each goal you have written down ask "What value does this express?" If you have a goal to, say, become a director at your company and your top value is freedom, you may have a conflict of interest if becoming a director will replace some of your freedom with late nights completing hundred-page reports and a leash to your cell phone. If you find goals that are not in alignment with your values, notice where the conflict is and if there is a different goal that would better align. As with goals we go after for someone else, goals we set because we think we should always lead to frustration.

Toward the end of my corporate career, there was one morning during my commute when every cell in my body wanted to drive past my freeway exit and not stop until I got far, far away. Even though I worked for a great company and had success in the traditional sense, my work didn't fit with who I saw myself to be. I struggled back and forth between conforming and taking a risk to live out my values.

The values you place importance on are not going anywhere. You can structure your life to ignore who you are, but the pull toward your values will always be there. The farther you get from your values, the more stressed you will be. For example, if you hold honesty as a high value but you lie, the guilt that you feel is the stress between your value of honesty and the story you've concocted. Save yourself the stress. Figure out a way to fit your goals around your values.

Step 4: Identify Small Actions

Phillip and I spent our eighth anniversary on the shores of Lake Tahoe. Just a few months earlier I had become a full-time entrepreneur, and, like most entrepreneurs, I was confused. I felt that I was being pulled in ten different directions and wasn't sure where I should put my energy. Most of our conversations those days were about what I could be doing in my business and this trip was no exception. After I laid out all of the options for the umpteenth time as Phillip patiently listened, he asked me "what is the *one* thing you think you should put your full focus on?" My answer came quickly. "I want to write a book." Under the backdrop of my treasured Sierra, I knew that a book was my next step. But a whole book, yikes. I spent a few months in panic mode feeling like there was too much to do, so I didn't do anything.

Things only started moving forward when I gave myself small daily actions to take that, in total, added up to this book. The first day I started on the book, all I had to do was come up with some tentative chapters. Eventually, the task was to write the first section of one chapter. As the process moved on things came together more quickly, and I found a publisher, started interviewing the amazing women featured, and eventually wrote the last word you will read in this book.

Some goals will be easy to schedule, like calling the skydiving company and making a reservation; but others will require you to plan things out. For goals that are longer range, write down small things you can do to move in that direction. This is especially helpful if your illness means that you may spend some days with little or no energy. By breaking down your goals small enough, you will be more likely to do a small thing on a day that you don't feel great rather than continuing to put your life on hold because starting your blog seems too big a task. Today, just pick the name of the blog.

Working with Your Body to Meet Your Goals

If you have always been a productive person, illness can push every button you have around needing to accomplish things. Our sense of self-worth comes from being able to recite all that we crossed off our to-do list in a day. Having to leave your job, take extra naps, or go to bed at 7:00 P.M. can make you feel like you're not doing your part. We beat ourselves up for the way our body is letting us down.

I have had numerous mental arguments about why I feel tired. My body is coping with a lot and has every reason to need extra rest, the lab tests concur and show that I have kidney disease–related anemia, but I sometimes fall into the trap of labeling myself as lazy or unmotivated. Sometimes I even secretly think I'm letting my husband down when, let's be honest, I'm just letting myself down.

Adding goals on top of the adjustment you're making to living with an illness can be tricky. Balance is the lesson every patient needs to learn. The technique that I use to address this I learned from Mary Kay. I was asked to give a presentation to a group of Independent Beauty Consultants and in preparation for the event I read Mary Kay's biography titled *Miracles Happen*.[6] Each day Mary Kay, who grew her company to more than $1 billion in sales and one million consultants worldwide, fifteen zeros combined, would make a list of six items to accomplish each day. That's it . . . just six! Before she began her workday, she would list the six most important things she needed to do and put them in priority order. Mary Kay would tackle the first thing on her list until that was finished and then move on to the next. If she only got through item number four, items five and six would become one and two the next day.

We live fragmented lives with the Internet, smartphones, and television. There is always a distraction around, and the stress of getting through a whole day and feeling like you didn't get anything done is annoying. Creating a small, manageable, daily task list helps you keep focused on your goals, which ultimately supports your values—much preferred to having your mind jump from here to there without getting anything done.

_____

6 Mary Kay, *Miracles Happen: The Life and Timeless Principles of the Founder of Mary Kay Inc.* (New York: HarperCollins, 1994), 82–84.

Mary Kay's magic number was six, but yours may be lower based on your level of health and how small you make the tasks on your list. "Clean the house" could be an item or "dust one photo" could be an item; that is up to you. It will take some experimenting, but eventually you'll settle into the right amount of to-do items in a day.

There is almost no better feeling than sliding your pen through something you accomplished that day, even if the only item on your list was to move from your bed to the couch. And we have all had those days.

A Conversation with Charity Sunshine Tillemann-Dick, Opera Singer, Idiopathic Pulmonary Hypertension and Double-Lung Transplant Survivor

Charity Sunshine Tillemann-Dick was diagnosed with idiopathic pulmonary hypertension (PH) and endured two double-lung transplants. She is an American-born soprano who has performed on the most prestigious stages across America, Europe, and Asia. Visit her at: *www.charitysunshine.com.*

"I was a nominally healthy person until I was diagnosed with PH [pulmonary hypertension] when I was twenty. I think I probably had PH for a very long time. It's chronically difficult to diagnose. When I was a little girl, I remember playing soccer, and long distances were almost impossible for me to run. It didn't matter how much I worked out at the gym. I always use to think I just must be lazy. Then I had four fainting episodes within a year. They were incredibly frightening, and I remember getting on my knees one night and just praying, saying, 'Dear God what is happening to me? If I'm

OK please, please just let me know, please just let me know that I'm all right, that everything is going to be OK and that I am just being paranoid, and please just let me know if in fact everything is OK.'"

Charity opened up her Bible looking for an answer. "I was really hoping that I'd get one of those happy stories in the Bible that everything is OK. Instead I got one of those terrible stories in the Old Testament about a king whose army was at war, and he told the Lord that if he let him win he would sacrifice whoever came to his room next, and in came his virginal favorite daughter who was the picture of virtue and goodness. It said that he wished he had been dead so he didn't have to follow through on it. I told my mother, and I started sobbing. I said, 'Mom, something's wrong with me.' I was diagnosed with PH about five months later."

PH is a thickening in the pulmonary veins, which caused the right chamber of Charity's heart to work harder to oxygenate her blood. The result is what she affectionately refers to as the "reverse Grinch effect": her heart grew three and a half sizes too big. This was the beginning of a long journey through two double-lung transplants that took her to the edge of life and to the height of her career. Charity's goals as a singer provided superhuman drive, multiple times, to blow past the obstacles PH was putting in her path.

"One thing I saw very quickly is that there are a lot of people whose life and whose existence is kind of defined by their disease, and I understand that to a certain extent. I understand that our experiences change us, but I was determined that this disease wasn't going to get in the way of me accomplishing what I had always wanted to accomplish. It was not going to get in the way of me singing. I felt that music was the gift, somehow music was the thing that I had been put here to share."

Charity has had to overcome several obstacles to stay committed to that gift. The first was the advice of a doctor. "There was a top specialist very early on who was adamant with me that I needed to stop singing, and that it would kill me if I didn't. I did a lot of research, and I didn't find anything to back up what she said. Even though she was an amazing doctor who had done a lot for my condition, I needed to find out what was going to help me survive this experience not only physically but emotionally, spiritually, and intellectually. I felt that singing was a really important part of maintaining my own humanity."

Knowing she was committed to music, Charity sought out a doctor who would support her decision to sing. That is when she met Dr. Reda Girgis of Johns Hopkins. "He understands that quality of life isn't just about being alive, even though being alive is a huge gift; he knew that for people to be happy in their lives they had to do things that made them happy. He was very supportive of me in my career. When I had professional opportunities in Europe, Asia, and the Middle East, he supported me. He'd say, 'Look, if you get worse you need to come back. But as long as you're doing all right, as long as your numbers are even and your physical activity isn't being impaired, you can continue.'"

Charity's love for music started early. "I went to go see *Hansel and Gretel* when I was four years old. It was amazing. I was in love; it was so beautiful. I wanted to sound just like the girl who sang Gretel. She had a particularly stunning voice." After a detour that involved studying politics and economics in college, Charity recommitted to her passion of music, which she says is "the purest form of communication." She attended the Franz Liszt Academy of Music in Budapest, "one of the best conservatories in Europe." Her career was just getting off the ground when she got the PH diagnosis.

For Charity, managing PH with diet and medication required inconceivable amounts of discipline and precision. For instance, the amount of sodium in a simple peanut butter and jelly sandwich could have sent her to the intensive care unit.

After Charity's father died unexpectedly, the grief over her loss and hectic travel schedule caused her PH to quickly progress. The only treatment that would ensure her survival was a double-lung transplant. Fortunately, the wait for the first set of lungs was less than a day.

Her first transplant surgery took thirteen and a half hours, during which she flatlined twice. She remained in a coma for five weeks afterward. With tenacity and perseverance, she miraculously recovered her health and her voice less than a year after she received her new set of lungs.

Her second transplant was a big surprise. "I got to a year and I had no rejection. It looked like things would probably be fine for quite awhile." Yet in November 2010, Charity caught a cold, which made her immune system ramp up, resulting in chronic rejection. "I knew that I was probably going to need another transplant for a year before I actually got it. I got to the point in July 2011 where it was really difficult for me to do anything. It was really difficult for me to walk, and, inexplicably and kind of remarkably, between July and my transplant I performed in seven cities. I would drive with my mom, who is amazing, kind of catatonic in the car. We [would] go to the hotel and I would sit there on oxygen and eat whatever I could. They would wheel me to the car, drive us over, and then wheel me to the stage. I'd try to stand up and I'd sing with the orchestra. Remarkably everything came out like it was supposed to come out, even though it was difficult for me to carry on a conversation." It was during that trying time that Charity fulfilled her dream of premiering alongside a prestigious group of performers at Lincoln Center in New York City.

When asked what has been the most challenging aspect of her health, Charity's mind drifts back to less than a year ago. "Waiting for this last transplant was mind bogglingly difficult. I think about it and I don't know how I'm alive today. I really don't. It's really difficult to describe the challenge of breathing when your lungs really don't want to, but if you could imagine living for six months where you had to consciously think about every breath you took, it takes up a lot of brain power and it takes up a lot of physical energy. Every day you don't think it could get worse, and then it does."

It is astounding to hear Charity's powerful voice that belts out arias with stunning precision describe not being able to breathe. But she worked diligently to train her voice before the transplants and worked after to regain what she once described as the closest thing to transcendence.

Having seen Charity sing, I wanted to know her perspective from the stage. What is it like to sing as beautifully as she does? "When I sing beautifully, it is wonderful. Sometimes I don't have good days because I think 'boy, that was horrible.' But when my voice is working the way that it has the potential to it is an out-of-body experience; the planets align. People think you sing from your lungs, or from your diaphragm, or from your throat, or from your vocal cords. They're not right. It engages your entire body in a very meaningful way. If you're not aligned properly, if you're not breathing in the right way, if you're not supporting in the right way, if you're not standing in the right way, if your chin is in the wrong position, if you're trying to force it, it's not going to come out like it's supposed to. When I perform that exchange of pure sound, it's something that's so inexplicably fulfilling. I'm just so deeply grateful that I experienced it."

As she rehabs from successful double-lung transplant number two, she is using her passion to fuel her singing career once again. Though, this time, she has to look at her career from a different angle. Transplant patients have to take immunosuppressant drugs which make them very susceptible to colds and more serious infections. Already having gone through one rejection, Charity is extra vigilant to preserve her health. This involves reassessing her goals.

"At this point, I'm trying to figure out what's the right goal for me because you have to be aware of your limitations. I'm incredibly sensitive to germs. I'm trying to figure out whether I need to be on stage alone, or whether I can still do opera like I used to, or [if it is] too risky to be with an entire ensemble of singers. I think part of living a meaningful life is not forgetting your dreams but figuring out the way that you're meant to live them.

> We look at what other people are doing and we judge ourselves according to others' success, when the truth is, success is never a comparative thing.

"There are a lot of people who have very specific ideas of what success means: 'success is twelve *New York Times* reviews [saying] how fantastic you are.' What I have realized is that I had to open myself to understand what success means for me because of my limitations. I may or may not have the traditional trajectory of my fellow students from conservatory. But just because we aren't singing in the same context doesn't mean that either of us is any more successful in what we're doing. We look at what other people are doing and we judge ourselves according to others' success, when the truth is, success is never a comparative thing. Look at yourself and your opportunities for growth and your limitations, and [see] how you can work with them, work around them.

"I realize I have to stop judging myself as harshly as I have. [I used to think] what did I do to deserve this? In my case, there was a huge amount of guilt that came with the rejection of my lungs, just racking my brain to think, 'What could I have done better? What did I do to cause this?'"

Charity's husband helped her realize that sometimes things go wrong despite your best intentions. She reflects now, "It's important to learn what we can from our mistakes, but not judge ourselves for them. That's the way to live with joy. I think the idea of living without regret is nice. The idea of living with joy is much better."

On June 19, 2012, I saw Charity perform for a packed house at the Moscone Center in San Francisco. She was the picture of elegance as she charmed the audience in a soft pink ensemble that included a glorious sequined skirt. To see her, you would never know the harrowing journey she has been on. Her joy lights up the room as she demonstrates just how resilient women can be.

HEALTH TIPS

- Focus on life goals in addition to your health.

- Setting goals provides motivation to follow care plans.

- Start with five value-based goals and take small actions toward them each day.

- Structure your day with a prioritized to-do list of no more than six items.

- Keep your goals flexible, and cultivate the patience to rest when you need to.

CHAPTER 4

Nourish Your Mind

I read an article once in the *Examiner* titled "GIRL, 5, GROWS NEW KIDNEYS!" in all capitals just like that. It goes on to profile Angel Burton, who was born with bilateral reflux that caused her kidneys to become damaged from urine flowing back to them, the same condition that damaged my kidney. When surgeons went in to fix her reflux, they found that she had grown two new kidneys right on top of the ones her congenital condition had damaged. Angel's story is astounding, and I am thankful that she has fully healed. I know that articles like this are intended to inspire hope and faith—who doesn't love a good "I overcame the odds" tale?—but for someone in the middle of illness, they can also subtly whisper the question, "Why haven't you healed yourself yet?"

As a child of the metaphysics movement, I used to dream that my speaking career would be centered on my miraculous healing. Something like: I inexplicably grew a second kidney and am now traveling to spread the good news that your faith in healing can cure all. I mistakenly connected the progression of disease in my body with there being something wrong at the core of who I am. The weight I placed on myself to become an anomaly was enormous, and, might I say, not very friendly. I have come to realize that my message is different. True healing comes from finding the compassion to unconditionally welcome ourselves exactly as we are.

Your New Friend

I talk to myself. All. Day. Long. My life is narrated by a high-pitched, sassy thing that has a tendency to blow things out of proportion. She jumps to conclusions. She questions my ability, and she second-guesses decisions I have already made. Do you have one of these self-talk companions too?

It can seem like the part of yourself that runs the mental dialogue is an enemy because it is her stories that are causing all of that worry. In truth, she has your best interests at heart. Really, she is scared. She wants desperately to protect you, to see you safe and happy and not make a fool out of yourself—that is why she won't let you tuck your pants into your socks anymore. She contemplates what will happen if the prednisone bloats you up and causes funky hair growth so that you will be ready, not because she likes to see you squirm.

Getting a diagnosis can send her into a frenzy. She anxiously wants to know how to help you heal. She throws out many ideas of what could help. Some are good ("a vacation may help you relax"); some are not so good ("if you weren't so darn negative you wouldn't be sick").

When we're sick, we say stupid things to ourselves. Messages that make us feel guilty or ashamed. Have you ever said anything like this to yourself?

- What use am I now?

- This is my karma coming back to bite me in the ass.

- So-and-so died of this.

- I am not thinking positive enough. I shouldn't cry, get angry, or feel depressed.

- I look like *$#%.

- I am a burden.

- Who will love me?

- I should not have eaten that/drunk that/ignored that.

- This is all my fault.

- This can only get worse.

Messages like this subtly, or not so subtly, communicate that you are not enough. The implication is that you are sick because you are not worthy of being well. This is a burden no friend would ever weigh you down with. A friend would hug you, stroke your hair, and tell you that you're beautiful. She would tell you that your illness makes you tough and that you are handling everything you've had to go through with exceptional grace.

> Remember, illness is just part of being human.

Remember, illness is just part of being human. It makes no judgments about "good" or "bad" people. It is an equal-opportunity offender. Being sick is a marathon, and as much support as you have around you from friends, family, and caregivers, you also have to support yourself. Becoming friends with yourself isn't as simple as "think positive" and all will be healed, as has been suggested numerous times in self-help books and the media.

The Self-Help Trap

The titles to some of today's most popular self-help books are nothing short of packaged miracles:

- *The Miracle of Mind Dynamics: Use Your Subconscious Mind to Obtain Complete Control Over Your Destiny* by Joseph Murphy

- *Creative Visualization: Use the Power of Your Imagination to Create What You Want in Your Life* by Shakti Gawain

- *The Power of Focus: How to Hit Your Business, Personal and Financial Targets with Absolute Certainty* by Jack Canfield

- *The Intention Experiment: Using Your Thoughts to Change Your Life and the World* by Lynne McTaggart

- *Awaken the Giant Within: How to Take Immediate Control of Your Mental, Emotional, Physical and Financial Destiny!* by Anthony Robbins

I am an avid self-help reader who has cracked open the books listed, plus many, many more, with the idea that somehow I would be able to live a dream life or at least grow that second kidney. There is a lot of pressure when you become ill to heal yourself. Everyone wants to believe in miracles. We want to know that if we become a better person, have deeper faith, or are able to control our thoughts, we could grow new organs or find ourselves in spontaneous remission.

I used to respond to that pressure by buying more books, assuming that I hadn't said my affirmations correctly, I hadn't released all of my limiting beliefs, or my inner child still had open wounds. I kept searching for the thing that would fix me, as if there was something wrong with not just my body but with who I was as a person. The marketing efforts around self-help make it seem like there is something hidden in those pages that, if I could just master it, would miraculously take all of my cares away. The message is that something is wrong with *you* if you have struggles in your life. That is a myth. The more you buy into the myth, the stronger the belief that you are not enough becomes. Illness shows us that life moves in cycles: flare-up, remission; pain, no pain; good day, bad day. Some days it goes your way and other days it doesn't—no matter how many books you read.

Of all the audiences that I have spoken with, when I ask the question "Has anyone here ever experienced a challenge?" I have yet to have an audience member not raise his or her hand. I haven't even run across someone who has said, "Well, I used to have problems until I read so-and-so's book, and now everything is perfect." The rough edges are part of life. They just are. That is something I willingly ignored. I bought into the marketing. I wanted to believe that I could manifest a cure. It gave me a false sense of control. It took a while to realize that the seven habits, four agreements, and five love languages were teaching how to get through the tough stuff, not how to make it disappear.

There are lots and lots of great self-help ideas out there. Things that can help you feel motivated and hopeful for a brighter future. Read and practice their techniques with appropriate expectations. Know that you are doing the best that you can. We are way, way more than enough, and it is time we start talking to ourselves as such.

Honor Your Emotions

One of the philosophies of the popular Law of Attraction movement is that our life flows from our thoughts. Good thoughts lead to a good life. This has led many women to begin diligently controlling their thoughts toward all things positive. If you have ever tried this, it is not easy. In fact, it can be a frustrating pursuit to go after each negative thought you have in fear that you must change it in order to have a happy and healthy life. The path typically starts with realizing just how many negative thoughts you have throughout the day and then trying to squash them like Whac-A-Mole and replace them with perfumed slogans about being perfect, whole, and gloriously complete. Your inner narrator is smarter than that. She knows when you're lying to yourself, and she is not going to believe that life is filled with light and vibrant health when you are tired, sick, or cranky.

When simply "thinking positively" does not work—when we get sick, stay sick, or even get worse—we tend to feel stressed and fearful about what is going on in our own minds. We shun our natural reactions in the face of trying to mentally turn things around. What ends up happening is that while you fake a smile and affirm that "divine energy is flowing through my body and healing my every cell," inside you feel terrified and out of control. A woman's emotional life is a rich mix of happy and sad, courageous and scared, grateful and resentful, and lots of other stuff she feels throughout the day. Some of the negative stuff will come with being sick. Honey, let it out. Be pissed if you're pissed. Be scared if you are scared. Be real. Pushing every negative emotion to the back burner means that those pots are still simmering. That does nothing to reduce your stress level or assist your healing. This does not mean that if you let your "positive guard" down you will cry all of the time. It does mean that while you may cry some, once the tears are dry you will feel more at ease and ready to take on the challenge in front of you.

Becoming your own supportive friend is not about convincing yourself that you are a glorious human being whose birthright is effervescent health. Friends listen

> Honey, let it out. Be pissed if you're pissed. Be scared if you are scared. Be real. Pushing every negative emotion to the back burner means that those pots are still simmering.

to the good stuff and the tough stuff. It is important to honor your full range of emotions.[7] Allow yourself time in your journal or with a trusted supporter to shake your fist at life every now and again.

VENTING

Turn to your journal when you need to get tough emotions out.

A New Approach: Honest Thinking

Dr. O. Carl Simonton coined the term "healthy thinking" as an alternative to "positive thinking" or "negative thinking."[8] Healthy thinking inspires hope by being consistent with the facts of reality. I adore this approach. To make the aim of this type of self-talk perfectly clear, I call it "*honest* thinking" because you are being completely honest with yourself. Rather than force yourself to be positive all of the time or get stuck in permanent negativity, think honestly to balance your emotions.

Take the statement "I am a burden" from earlier in the chapter. Can you know that statement is true? Or is it just an assumption you have made? Would your closest friend say that you are a burden?

Counteracting mental stress is about recognizing what is true at the moment. Not what you hope to be true, but what you know, what you can feel to be true.

---

7 Caren S. Fried, PhD, *Positive Thinking—Helpful or Harmful for Cancer Patients?: Thoughts on Living with Cancer* (New Jersey: New Beginnings, 1998).

8 O. Carl Simonton, MD, and Reid Henson, *The Healing Journey* (New York: Bantam Books, 1992), 56.

You will recognize truth when you feel relaxed about what you are thinking and saying. You will not feel like you are faking it or lying to yourself. Honest thinking is different from positive thinking in that it does not paint everything to be butterflies and rainbows.

A study led by psychologist Joanne Wood took a group of people and divided them into two groups: those with low self-esteem and those with high self-esteem.[9] Each group read positive statements such as "I am a loveable person." They found that positive thinking only helped the group that already had high self-esteem and actually made the group with low self-esteem—the group that needed the boost the most—feel worse. The headline of the report from BBC News was "Self-Help 'Makes You Feel Worse.'"[10]

The conclusion the report should have come to is that you can't lie to yourself to feel better; you have to believe what it is that you are telling yourself. The group with low self-esteem did not believe the statement "I am a loveable person" was true. The words they said were very different from what they actually thought and felt, which was probably "No, you are not a loveable person." They only reinforced their already existing negative self-image.

Have you ever tried to tickle yourself? Go on, try it now . . . under the arms or behind the knees. Can't do it? That is no surprise. It is really hard to manipulate ourselves. As with tickling, so it goes with changing thought patterns. Trying to convince yourself that life is perfect when it isn't is like trying to tickle yourself. It is impossible to trick ourselves when we know why we are doing it.

---

9   Joanne Wood, W. Q. Elaine Perunovic, and John W. Lee, "Positive Self-Statements: Power for Some, Peril for Others," *Psychological Science* (2009). doi: 10.1111/j.1467-9280.2009.02370.x.

10   "Self-Help Makes You Feel Worse" *BBC News* (July 2009). *news.bbc .co.uk/2/hi/8132857.stm*.

Building an internal friendship involves starting where you are at. If you do not feel great about yourself or your health, then yes, a statement such as "I have vibrant beauty and health" will do little more than make you want to crawl back into bed and put the covers over your head. Begin with talking to yourself about the positive aspects of what is true for you at this moment. Not what you *hope* to be true, but what you *know* to be true.

Honest thinking is more down-to-earth. More patient. More accepting. For example, if a positive thought about healing is "I will be cured in one year," an honest thought would be, "I do not know if I will be cured in one year, but I continue to take healthy actions." See the difference? Honest thinking points your focus in the direction of health without pretending that things are better than they might be.

If you find yourself in a cycle of worry or if you hear yourself being your enemy instead of your friend, do two things:

(1) Ask yourself if what you are thinking is true; and

(2) Replace your thought with the truth.

Worry is an assumption about something that has not yet happened. If you are worried that an upcoming scan will reveal the progression of your disease, ask yourself if you know that the disease has in fact progressed. The answer is no. Replace your worry with an honest thought such as: "I do not know what my scans will reveal, but I am committed to finding a path toward health."

There is no "right" way to do honest thinking. You do not need to say your thoughts into a mirror, write them down, or use any particular phrasing. Simply use your own style of speaking to yourself and hear the truth in what you are saying. The key is that the words you use should help you feel empowered. Here are some of my favorite honest thoughts about healing:

- The treatments I follow are helping my body heal.

- I choose to be patient with my body and my mind.

- I trust that I am guided toward the doctors and treatments that will restore my health.

- I choose to be thankful for my toes, feet, ankles, legs, knees . . . head, hair.

- I am grateful for my doctors and nurses.

- I am willing to take good care of myself.

- I have the potential to heal.

- The medicine I take knows exactly what to do in my body to help me get better.

- I listen to and trust my intuition to guide me toward healing.

If the above statements do not feel true for you, adjust them until they are believable. It can help to add the words "potential," "choose," or "willing" to statements that feel untrue to adjust them for where you are at. For instance, "The treatments I follow help my body to heal" would become "The treatments I follow *have the potential to* help my body heal."

HONEST THINKING MANTRA

Write down a mantra that you believe in, a statement that makes you feel empowered as you repeat it.

One of my favorite mantras comes from Meredith Israel Thomas (see chapter 1). As she would say, "I am going to kick cancer's ass!" Choose an honest thinking mantra for yourself. It can be one from the previous list or a statement that especially resonates with you from a spiritual text or other inspirational source. Memorize your mantra and repeat it often. The more often you remind yourself of what is true, the quicker you will build internal support and self-compassion.

I Can

You give up a lot when you get a diagnosis. Those losses may include the freedom of your time, the freedom to eat what you want, or the freedom to travel where you wish. Loss is something we like to remind ourselves of.

A few years ago it became clear that I needed to give up eating meat because animal protein can be especially hard on the type of kidney damage I have. When I realized that I needed to make this change, the only thing I could focus on is what I'd be losing: meat lasagna, turkey at Thanksgiving, chicken tacos, and tuna fish sandwiches (best with pickles and cheddar on sourdough). My "I can't eat that" attitude made my cravings stronger, and becoming vegetarian felt very limiting, as if I would never be able to enjoy food again.

Would a friend remind you of all the things you will have to give up or miss out on because you need to concentrate on your health? Of course not. She would remind you of what you can still do, can still enjoy, and can still contribute.

After a few months cycling through eating meat and feeling guilty, I decided to focus only on what I *could* eat. When looking at a restaurant menu I would ask myself "What can I eat?" or "How can I order that to be vegetarian?" Meal planning at home would be the same. "How can I substitute for the meat in this recipe?" It took me a while to come up with a good substitute for the tuna sandwich, but the difference in my feelings of deprivation were like night and day when I started using the word "can" instead of "can't."

What losses do you need to stop focusing on in your own life? Where *can* you put your focus instead? If you cannot hike, can you take a drive in the mountains? If you cannot swim, can you enjoy the water on a boat? If you have to reduce the fat in your diet, can you find a healthier recipe for your favorite cheesy comfort food?

> The difference in my feelings of deprivation were like night and day when I started using the word "can" instead of "can't."

It is important to develop healthy mental habits to give yourself a break from thinking about your illness. The rest of this chapter details some of my favorite visualizations and ways to distract yourself in nourishing ways.

Take a Visual Vacation

Remember your first kiss. How does that moment come back into your awareness? Most likely, it is through a picture. You can visualize the scene—you see him lean in, you feel your eyes close, and your lips meet. Reliving this moment through pictures causes the feelings to bubble back up. Visualization is the art of using your imagination to lead yourself toward feelings of relaxation, safety, comfort, clarity, and joy.

You have probably practiced creating scenes of worry. I know that when I hear the *T* word, the first image in my mind is myself in a hospital bed. The idea of visualization is to consciously choose to spend some time imagining other more relaxing scenarios. By sinking your mind into images that create feelings of comfort, you are reducing stress. You give your body a break, boost your immune system, and lower your blood pressure. My favorite visualizations for feeling relaxed and taking a break from the frustrations of illness are below. The first two are based on exercises found in Shakti Gawain's book *Creative Visualization*. She presents them in her book as: "Creating Your Sanctuary"[11] and "Meeting Your Guide."[12]

Visualization 1: Find Your Sacred Space

Think of your favorite, most relaxing, most enjoyable place to be. It could be a cherished vacation spot, an inviting chair in a quiet corner of your home, or anything else that calms your spirit.

When my family would vacation in the High Sierras, the mornings were always my favorite. The sun lit up the mountaintops with pink splendor, the air was crisp and cool, and there was always a softly gurgling stream nearby. As I walked the campsite, I could hear my sneakers crunch on the rocks and leaves below. It was a place where I never felt separate from the moment. I always felt included, connected, and grateful.

Once you have your space in mind, close your eyes and picture yourself there. Notice everything—how it looks, how it sounds, and especially how you feel. Just stand for a moment in your space. Take it in. Once you have absorbed the details of your surroundings, adjust the space to make it even more inviting. Add a chair, turn a light on, raise the sun a bit, bring in your favorite book or journal, pour yourself something delicious to drink, invite your favorite pet, or add some flowers.

---

11 Shakti Gawain, *Creative Visualization: Use the Power of Your Imagination to Create What You Want in Your Life* (California: New World Library, 2002), 82–83.

12 Ibid., 84–86.

Keep making adjustments and noticing how you feel. Once you experience a feeling of deep calm and serenity, take some time to enjoy being in your space. Allow it to soak into every inch of your mind and body. When you feel ready, you can move on to another visualization or open your eyes.

The space you have created is a place you can go to just by closing your eyes. You can begin or end your day there, or you can use your space to contemplate decisions, let go of stress, or do anything else that comes to mind. It can be a good place to go to while in a CT scan, MRI, or hospital bed, too. It's your private anytime vacation.

Visualization 2: Meet Your Higher Self

Your higher self is the part of you that is calm, cool, and collected. She is a wise and confident woman who can help you navigate life, and it is about time you met her.

Close your eyes and relax. Picture yourself in your sacred space designed in the exercise above. Take some time to reexplore your space and enjoy the vibe there. When you are ready, picture a figure walking toward you from off in the distance. This is the fuzzy, intangible, wise, spiritual side of yourself. As she comes closer, her appearance will come into view. She may look like you or she may not. She might be translucent or glowing. She might not even be human; she could be an animal or any other being. Observe her walking closer and take in the details of her face, her body, and her spirit. Invite her to join you. You can speak with her as you would anyone else. She has a lot to offer you, and she is there to support you in any way you ask of her. Some questions you might consider asking her are:

• What is the next step?

- What is most important right now?

- What do I need to focus my attention on?

- What do I need to understand in this situation?

- What is important for me to do to heal?

Once you have asked your questions, sit quietly and listen. Your higher self may not speak in words; you may get a feeling or moment of intuition that nudges you toward your answer. Once you feel your conversation is complete, thank your higher self (you can even hug it out), and begin to focus your attention on your breath as you bring your mind back to full awareness.

Visualization 3: Ahhh . . . Love

Good health days are synonymous with more love. If you are having a day of great energy, clear focus, and low pain, are you not more in love with those around you? If you are celebrating a victory, does it not feel amazing to hug and laugh and smile with the people you love? When you are afraid of your future health outcomes, I would bet that part of your fear includes being taken from your family or not being able to care for someone you love. The more people I talk to, the more I am convinced that everything comes back to love—wanting to give love and receive love. This visualization transports you to the woozy feeling we all crave.

Close your eyes and relax. In your mind's eye, picture yourself with someone you love. It could be a spouse, your children, or a cherished member of your extended family or friends. Notice where you are—are you sharing a meal? On vacation? In your home? Focus on your loved one's face and allow yourself to feel utterly and completely head over heels in love. Just like the first time you fell for him or her. In this groovy state of love, expand the feeling by including touch. You can hold hands, hug, dance, cuddle, or even do the horizontal tango. Allow all of this person's energy and love to enter your heart. Feel the surge of love spread throughout your body. Bask in the sweetness. Once you have overwhelmed yourself with the bliss of love, return to the room you are in by shifting your focus toward your breathing. Conclude by opening your eyes.

Visualization 4: Shining Sun

This is a personal favorite. It is very simple. Relax as you have done in the other visualizations. Picture yourself standing below the sun on a gorgeous, clear day. Tilt your face toward the sun and feel the warmth of the sun's rays bathe your entire body. Try smiling during this visualization to up the joy factor as you commune with the sun. Allow the bright, brilliant light to wash your body of any aches and pains, any worries and fears. Continue as long as you wish.

The Process

Research has shown that attaining goals is as much about anticipating the challenges in the process as it is about excitedly anticipating the outcome.[13] When you are dealing with a health challenge, there may be some unpleasant tests, treatments, and side effects between you and your goal of health. Visualizing medical procedures can help mentally prepare you for any rough patches.

When I was young, and not-so-young, I would go for an annual radiology test called a voiding cystourethrogram

---

13 Peter M. Gollwitzer and Gabriele Oettingen, "The Role of Goal Setting and Goal Striving in Medical Adherence." In *Medical Adherence and Aging. Social and Cognitive Perspectives,* D. C. Park and L. L. Liu (eds.), Washington, DC: American Psychological Association, 2007, 23–47.

(VCUG) to check my kidney reflux. It is an awful test, and I pray you never have to endure it. They insert a catheter, fill your bladder up with a radiocontrast solution, and watch on a screen for the moment when the solution escapes your bladder and goes back up toward your kidneys. (That's the reflux.) Once your bladder is fuller-than-full, they ask you to urinate on the X-ray table to see if constricting the bladder exacerbates the reflux. I have never been able to pee on a table in a room filled with techs. That doesn't mean that they don't try to make you pee by turning on the faucet and even pouring water over your legs. I would scream and cry every year until they let me go use the toilet. Once when I was seven years old, I was determined to hold it together. I mentally walked myself through the procedure to prepare for what was coming. The test was horrific as always, but I was beaming with pride when I came out of there tear-free. I have used this same visualization each time I have a VCUG, and I'm happy to report that I didn't cry when I endured it again last summer.

Visualization 5: Processing an Event You're Nervous About

Before you begin the visualization, determine how you want to feel during and after your medical treatment. Relax by closing your eyes and taking a few deep breaths. Imagine yourself calmly entering the treatment room. Mentally walk through the procedure as it has been described to you by medical staff. During the treatment, picture yourself being open to healing. Let go and allow trust to wash over your body. Imagine the procedure being smooth and successful. Feel the way you had chosen prior to the visualization. Open your eyes and bring your new confidence to your procedure with you.

This style of visualization can be used for all sorts of processes: making dietary choices, having a great workout, completing a project, overcoming an obstacle, laying out your daily routines, or anything else you come up with.

Visualization Tips

Your imagination can create scenes of elation, celebration, and peace. Here are my best tips for upping the feeling factor of your visualizations:

- Preplan the details of what you will be visualizing. When I am not quite sure what I will be imagining, my mind jumps around trying to change and adjust the scene, never really allowing me to enjoy it. If you are picturing a nice dinner out, decide who will be there, where you are eating, what is on the menu, what beverage you will enjoy, and which dress you will dazzle in.

- Smile. Our bodies are great communicators, and physically smiling will entice you to emotionally smile also. You can often find me grinning from ear to ear at what my mind has come up with.

- Try moving. OK, I know this sounds odd, but rocking while you visualize can, *swoosh*, completely immerse your mind in your visualization. After I begin a visualization session, I will gently rock in my chair from side to side or backward to forward. No rocking chair necessary, just lightly bounce off the pillows behind you. You may find that this movement takes on a life of its own; just go with it. I believe there's something about moving that occupies the conscious thinking mind and allows the imagination to take over.

- If you have a hard time visualizing, look at old photo albums to recall fond memories. This can be a dreamy way to spend an afternoon when lying low and resting.

* * *

Now that we have talked about how to become a friend to ourselves through compassionate self-talk and visualizing nourishing scenes, the next step is to create a toolbox of distraction so that when pain, worry, or fear becomes intense, you have some ways to change the subject.

Distraction

Hospitals are sterile places. Their stark white walls make the monitors and IV drips stand out even more. They are not often associated with music.

I was seven when I found myself back in the hospital with another bout of pneumonia. I spent most of my days watching shows like *The Mickey Mouse Club* and *The Electric Company* while the antibiotics did their thing. My mom and I would joke that my pulse oximeter, which makes your finger glow red, was my way to communicate with E.T. On one special afternoon, my dad visited with his guitar. Looking at me the way only a father can as he takes in his daughter and her pain, he sang to me. He played Bette Midler's "The Rose," and we cried. It was the only thing to do. That memory sticks out to me more than the oxygen mask, the shots, and the breathing treatments. In fact, the medical stuff and pain fade into the background. The sweet moments are what stay with you. There was only one song that would do for the father-daughter dance at my wedding.

Stress diminishes your ability to think clearly. That is why it is so much easier to eat a bag of chips or zone out in front of the TV than it is to think of healthier alternatives, such as walking or calling an old friend when you are tired or emotionally drained. Now is the time, before you are in a cycle of worry or have a headache, to determine how you will distract yourself from the immediacy of your discomfort.

DISTRACTIONS

Create a go-to list of your favorite distractions for implementation when pain or worry becomes intense.

Get your creativity flowing and see how many nourishing distractions you can surround yourself with or prepare to have on hand when you need them. Here are a few suggestions to get you started:

- New artwork. Take your favorite honest thoughts from earlier in the chapter and paste them all over your house. A note on the fridge that says "I care about my body" just might change your eating habits. They can be decorated with stickers, printed in vibrant colors, or crafted any way you like. Channel your inner kindergartener and let her go to town. Crayons and markers are a must.

- Get outside. There is something about trees, sun, fresh air, flowers, and water that calls to joy and pulls it forth. If it is a sunny day, go for a walk or a drive to a place with more trees than cement. If it is raining outside, sit by a window and drink a cup of something steamy as you watch the rain. Plant a garden or a flowerbed. Dig your hands into the earth, get muddy, watch for your favorite birds, marvel at a glimpse of a deer. With all of the "smart" technology out there, our connection to the earth gets buffered. Go explore in any way you can.

Even just wandering a plant nursery can brighten your day.

- Revamp the iPod. Create a playlist of your favorite songs. Ones that make you jump and dance, smile and sing, or maybe just relax and groove. And why not dance while you do the dishes or clean? Think back to the music that marked moments of celebration or peace in your life. Music can be especially calming during medical procedures.

- Overhaul your library. What you read counts, too. Ditch the gossip magazines for higher-grade eye candy. Pick something funny, romantic, inspirational, informative, or imaginative to fill your mind with. Get recommendations from your friends, a local librarian, or the bestsellers list to choose your next read. You might want to try revisiting some of your most cherished books from when you were young. *The Giving Tree* by Shel Silverstein always makes me feel grateful.

- Movie night. Need I say more? Pop some salt-and-oil-free popcorn and laugh yourself silly. Study after study has shown that laughter can act as medicine. Movie night has always been an integral part of my healing process. I distinctly remember laughing at *The Money Pit* until my stitches literally hurt after an operation. Essential ingredient? Funny!

- Watch TV. Ahh . . . the boob tube. Television can be a great escape from pain and illness. But tread lightly, dear one. It can quickly become a crutch to escape from your thoughts and life. Television changes your brain waves so that you internalize the messages you are watching. When you find that it is becoming your only pastime and that your energy wanes when you turn it on, it is time to take a break and feast your eyes on something less hypnotizing. In moderation, and with the use of our modern nifty DVRs, selectively choose what you want to watch, record it, and stick to your plan. In periodic doses, TV can be fun and bust a stitch or teach you something new.

Since you have decided to be the owner of your life, you get to decide what sort of friend you are going to be to yourself. Manage that responsibility with care. Your stress level and immune system will thank you for it.

A Conversation with Lauren Nastasi, Mother, Blogger, and Crohn's Pioneer

Lauren Nastasi is on the frontier of coping with Crohn's disease. She is a blogger and mother spreading the benefits of diet and attitude to manage her health. Visit her at: *www.gingeristhenewpink.blogspot.com.*

"That's when I ended up in the ICU and almost in cardiac arrest with blood transfusions, and just really sick. I had to get a hold [of myself] and say, 'OK, you have this disease; they have told you that it's a lifetime sentence. You're just going to have to figure out how to deal with it.' I changed my diet and changed my attitude, relaxed more, and did more exercises to help myself be aligned."

Lauren Nastasi had been healthy her whole life, but when she was twenty-two, things changed. "I was feeling sick out of nowhere. I actually thought that I needed more fiber or something; I wasn't going to the bathroom. I took a laxative and that night everything came out. I was bleeding and really, really ill. I thought maybe I had food poisoning; I had had Chinese food that night and [thought] 'Oh, no!' I didn't really eat meat at that time, so I was cursing at tofu, like, what the heck?"

As she coped with her mysterious symptoms, she confided in her mom that she was seeing blood in her stool. Her mom, obviously concerned, urged her to see a doctor. After a trip to the ER Lauren was told she had ulcerative colitis and was put on medication to ease her symptoms. "They put me on drugs, and it actually got better. And then it got worse again. I was fed up with the whole thing. I didn't believe in medicine. I didn't take Tylenol to begin with, and now I was taking twelve pills a day. It was really, really hard for me to wrap my head around that, and I said to my husband, 'Well, I'm not going to take the medicine and just let my body heal itself.'"

That is when Lauren ended up in the ICU. Ultimately she was diagnosed with Crohn's disease, an inflammatory bowel disorder that causes inflammation in the digestive tract typically centered in the intestines. Knowing that Crohn's would be with her for a long time, she took charge to figure out the best diet and routine for her body. She started walking a path to become better acquainted with her digestive system and the connection between her mind and body. This prompted her to become closer friends with herself.

Lauren was told by her medical team that "'there's no correlation between diet and the disease so you can go out and eat whatever you want. You can eat hamburgers and fries, this and that. It has nothing to do with how sick you get.'" This didn't sit well. Lauren thought, "Come on, *stomach* disease, how is food not related to it? I did a lot of trial and error. I knew eating plain stuff was making me worse, so I started cutting out eggs, and then chicken, and then it came down to what was left." She was careful to pace her dietary changes. "I took it very slow because I was not about to kick myself into a flare-up and be in the hospital again."

After growing up in an Italian household with lots of meat and cheese, Lauren did something dramatic out of compassion to care for her body. "I eventually became a vegan. No dairy, no meat, no eggs, nothing, and I found that I felt best when I ate that way, surprisingly, because you wouldn't think raw foods would be good for the stomach. But for some reason, I guess the enzymes and whatnot actually helped me out a lot." She eventually also cut out gluten. While going gluten-free was the "hardest thing," Lauren sees the benefits. "Once in awhile if I even have something little I'll know right away, and [I think] 'oh, I shouldn't have done that! It's not worth it!' It's just not worth it in the end."

Managing Crohn's disease is about minimizing flare-ups and coping with them when they inevitably happen. While diet plays a big role in controlling symptoms, there is a very real connection between the body and our mental and emotional states. From learning about Lauren, I knew that she had explored this relationship in depth as she reinvented her relationship with her body to work around Crohn's. I asked her, "Do you see a connection between how stressful your life is at any moment and what your body is reflecting to you?" Lauren didn't hesitate. "Oh, definitely, definitely." Lauren recalled when she gave birth to her daughter. "I had an emergency C-section. The cord was wrapped around her neck, and she swallowed meconium. She was in the NICU for seven days. Right after that I definitely had a flare-up. Since then, it's been a constant battle because I have a child now, so I'm always a little stressed, a little on edge!"

Lauren has worked with her outlook and attitude to minimize her symptoms. "I think I've trained myself, my brain, because at first I used to cry every day, 'why do I have this disease? Why me? What did I do wrong?' Eventually, I had to change my mindset. It was almost like it clicked in my head, 'If you're happy and everything else in your life is happy, then who cares about this little thing?'" When she is worried or her "monkey brain's going," Lauren continually reminds herself "'this is nothing. You'll get through this. Tomorrow's a new day; it's not worth getting sick over.' If you're negative, it's going to make you sick. When I get upset, it starts to trigger my Crohn's. There's no point in being upset or being negative about anything, it's not going to do any good to be negative. Being positive has helped me feel like I have a blessed, beautiful life."

Lauren has turned toward the positive, but she recognizes that sometimes she needs to let more painful emotions out, and she works with those emotions in a focused and constructive way. "Once in awhile I do let myself cry, obviously. You've got to let it out sometimes. Journaling definitely helps, just getting the emotions out, even if I have to spend a few minutes venting to my husband, or whatever. I can't let myself dwell on it. I've got to give myself an allotted time period. [I'll tell my husband] 'OK, I'm going to tell you everything that went bad in my day, and then I'm not going to talk about it the rest of the day.'"

With so many lifestyle adjustments, I asked Lauren how Crohn's changed her relationship with herself. "It's been seven years; I would definitely say I'm at a completely different place than I used to be. I used to worry a lot and let every little thing bother me. When I see people that let the little things bother them, I can't understand them. [I think] 'why are you letting this bother you? There's nothing that worrying is going to do to fix it; it's no big deal.' On a big scale [Crohn's is] very small, and that's what I feel about my disease. I feel like this is minuscule compared to everything else that I have in my life. There's no point in letting that [Crohn's] ruin everything else in my life. That's definitely different from what I used to think!"

Lauren has gathered a solid toolkit to foster her new-found outlook and keep stress at bay; I wanted to know what her new self-care routines were. "I pray every night. I talk to God, pray for other people around me, thank Him, and express gratitude for everything that I have. I also like to do visualizations of my intestines. I try to imagine white, glowing light around my stomach. Especially when I meditate, I think about light coming in from maybe the sky, coming into my stomach, glowing, and healing. Everything just looks perfect and pink and not inflamed—whatever it really looks like! Visualization definitely helps keep positivity in my life. It is not helpful to think all the time 'oh my gosh, I'm sick. I'm diseased. This is all messed up inside me!' When I go for a colonoscopy, I don't like them to show me the pictures of the results because I don't want to know what it looks like. I just want to have this vision in my head that everything is healing and going right."

In addition to mental exercises, Lauren has a few go-to's for physically distracting herself from stress. "I find that lifting weights is nice and makes you feel strong when you're feeling weak. It definitely changes your mindset. I do yoga and walk with [my daughter] to the park in her stroller. I find that being outside, hiking, being in the sun, anything like that helps. With yoga, the breathing exercises help to clear my mind. A good workout, something about sweating, it clears your mind of anything."

Like everyone, Lauren can fall behind on her self-care sometimes, but she is quick to recognize the benefits of consistency and makes time to stay dedicated to her health. "I'll fall off the wagon for a few weeks, and then I'll start to notice the tension in my body, maybe I'll get a backache or my stomach will start bothering me, and I [realize], you know what? It's worth keeping up with.

The motivation of feeling better, knowing in my head that I'm going to feel better if I do this, [encourages me to] just do it, make the time, carve out five minutes. It's worth it!"

In the end, Crohn's has changed her view of life. "I try to live day by day. Crohn's isn't a death sentence, but you never know what tomorrow will bring. I could be perfect today and then tomorrow be bedridden. When I'm feeling good, I try to enjoy every moment I have that I'm healthy and not on the couch. I like to do everything that I want to do. If I want to go for a hike, I go for a hike. If I want to go for dinner in the city, my husband and I go for dinner in the city. We try to do things and make the good days good and memorable."

Today, Lauren has posted a picture online of the fresh green juice she is sharing with her daughter. In that one glass is the journey to develop the self-care and compassion of the best friend a girl could have.

HEALTH TIPS

- Become your own friend by speaking kindly to yourself.

- Take the pressure off, let go of miraculous expectations.

- Use *honest* thinking to combat stressful worries.

- Use visualization to relax and refocus.

- Surround yourself with positive, nourishing literature, music, and programming.

CHAPTER 5

Reassess the Space You Keep

I tied a lavender sachet to the cage door in preparation for what I thought would be five very rough weeks. Our dog Abbey was having ACL surgery. The vet's instructions were that Abbey would need to be caged for five weeks to allow her knee to heal properly. The only time she could get out of her cage was for a slow walk outside on a leash to potty.

We never crate trained Abbey. She was four months old and already potty trained when we adopted her from the Humane Society. From night one, she has slept in our bed, all roly-poly on her back in between our pillows, inevitably with her rear in one of our faces. Yes, we are pushovers to her impossibly sweet eyes and soft, snuggly fur. Abbey is also an energetic dog. People find it hard to believe that she is ten given the way she races around our house, making sharp turns to cut back under the dining room table as we chase after her; hence, the torn ACL.

Abbey also has a sister, Emma, a fun-loving mutt who gets her all riled up. I could not imagine how Abbey was going to have the patience to live in a cage for five whole weeks.

We got a large cage and a pad to line the bottom covered in ultrasoft microfiber. I put a towel and another blanket against the back wall for added comfort. I tied on the lavender sachet in the hope that calming aroma-therapy would soothe her nerves while she was healing.

It is heartbreaking to have your pet go through major surgery. You want so badly to explain that the pain will benefit her in the long run. You want to ask how you can ease her discomfort and have her understand that you are so sorry she has to go through this.

The first evening was the hardest. She had to wear a cone collar inside the cage and she softly whimpered throughout the night. Phillip and I took turns sleeping with our head at the edge of the cage so that she would know we were there. Emma even took a shift early in the morning guarding the cage while we got dressed for the day.

For the entire five weeks, Abbey was an amazingly good girl. She intuitively understood that she needed to heal. She began to see her cage as a place of rest and refuge. She willingly went inside each time we came back from potty breaks and slept calmly most of the day and night. She let me ice her knee and allowed Phillip to stretch it when it was time for physical therapy. Emma even understood that Abbey needed the cage and didn't coerce her to play at any point.

The vet said she healed beautifully; he was impressed by how she recognized her limitations and tolerated the cage. Abbey taught me a lot about acceptance in those five weeks. She demonstrated a deep understanding of what healing required and honored what her body needed most.

After the five weeks were up, she never went in the cage or wanted to be anywhere near it again.

Cater to Your Senses

Many times the space we keep, mainly our home and office, caters to our schedules. Dishes fill the sink while we rush off to work, our clothes drape over a chair because we're too tired to put them away, and papers quickly accumulate into a leaning tower.

What if our environment catered to our senses instead of our schedule? Sight, hearing, taste, touch, and smell are how we experience the world. Through these senses information is delivered to our brain, and it makes certain assessments about what is going on around us and how we should react to it, including how stressed we should be. The senses are the messengers of stress. When you look around and see muddy paw prints on the floor, hear a blaring television, or smell the trash that needed to be emptied two days ago, do you not feel more on edge?

When you're stressed, energy is diverted away from your immune system to address the cause of the stress. Your health needs that energy back. Structuring your environment to cater to your senses means creating a space that renews your energy instead of depleting it.

The philosophy behind building a temple is to dissolve the barrier between the world and the divine. A temple's purpose is to assist with quieting the mind and opening the spirit. The use of art, religious symbols, simplicity, light, shadow, and connection with nature blur the stresses of daily life and heighten the sense of energy within.

I am a realistic person and know that you're not going to keep your house spotless or your office completely organized. I'm not perfect either. But I do suggest that you create a few spaces in your life that are sacred. Personal temples, if you will. Places that you can go to rest and feel at peace.

My temple for healing when I was young was our family room couch. At the first sign of being sick, my mom would piece together my temporary bed. The sheets were seventies wonders with brown and orange pinwheels on a white background; they would get tucked neatly around the cushions and the top would fold back over a few blankets. A TV tray was set up next to the couch for tissues, breathing devices, the remote, and a glass of fresh carrot and apple juice, my family's elixir for anything that ailed you. When the couch was ready, my mom would get me out of bed, and I'd move to the heartbeat of the house, ready to be nursed well.

When I don't feel well today, I still park myself on the couch; it doesn't even cross my mind to stay in bed. There is something comforting about returning to the traditions of my childhood. If I know my back is out or if I am sick, I'll gather my loot from bookshelves, the medicine cabinet, and the kitchen and park in the family room. (I wish I still had the sheets with the orange and brown pinwheels, though. They would make my healing temple complete.)

Think about which rooms in your home are the best for rest and relaxation, and which rooms you spend the most time in. These are the targets for your makeover. For me, the family room, my office, and the bedroom are the places that make me tranquil or cranky. In each room, tune in to your senses. Think about how the space makes you feel and what changes could create a true refuge.

Explore each sense to design an environment that preserves your energy and promotes health.

Sight

Sight is intimately connected with emotion. It is the sense that is predominant for most people, and because of that, sight is a powerful tool for decreasing stress. Tranquility in your visual environment becomes tranquility in your mind.

Clean It Up

Keeping your sacred spaces clean is one of the single most important tasks to create a place of rest. Clutter in our rooms clutters up our minds. If you don't have the energy or time to keep your space clean, split up the chores between family members or hire a cleaning service.

Just as when you have fifteen minutes notice before surprise guests arrive, there are lots of shortcuts you can take to create the appearance of cleanliness without actually "cleaning."

- Keep closet doors and drawers shut.

- Make the bed each morning.

- Gather scattered papers into one stack and place that stack out of view.

- Wipe down the sink and faucet with a rag after brushing your teeth and washing your face to avoid splatter marks.

- When you take your clothing off, hang it back up or put it in a concealed hamper right away.

- Straighten pillows and blankets on the couch.

- Wipe crumbs off the counter.

- If you have lots of medications, tissues, and other paraphernalia crowding your nightstand or coffee table, get a small tray to corral the things you need. You can also place a small wastebasket or bucket near you for trash.

These small steps create the appearance and mind-set of cleanliness without the symptom-exacerbating work of actually cleaning.

When you do have the energy, a weekend of spring-cleaning can do wonders to refresh your mind, body, and spirit. My rule of thumb is: if I don't love it or need it, someone else will; donate it.

Redecorate

Once your space is picked up, add a few visual touches that are personally comforting.

- Cover your walls with family photos. There are a number of online services that will enlarge and print your photos on canvas for a reasonable price.

- Add indoor plants and flowers to your space.

- Light candles.

- Build a fire in the fireplace.

- Print out your favorite quotes and hang them around your room.

- Buy or create art for your walls.

- Add crystals or other objects of visual interest to shelves or the mantel.

- Include meaningful symbols of your faith.

Adjust the Lighting

Light is another way to create a relaxing environment. Consider opening your curtains to let the sun in during the day, and shutting them for restful sleep at night. Add nightlights for a soft glow. If you have trouble sleeping, a sleeping mask could be a true blessing, especially if your place of rest is in the hospital where monitors glow all night long. A personal lighting favorite of mine is twinkling Christmas lights any time of year. You can wrap them around houseplants and drape them over shelves or drapery rods.

Watch Something New

If you are tired of watching the same old reruns on television, pop in a meditation DVD or search for a meditation program through your cable's On Demand service. There are a number of programs that play soft music and show images of nature. Watching a nature DVD for just ten minutes has been shown to significantly decrease stress.[14]

Step Outside

Getting out of the house is another fantastic way to refresh your spirit by changing what you look at. You could take a day-trip to the ocean, the mountains, or your favorite small town. Researchers Clare Cooper Marcus and Marni Barnes have shown that 95 percent of people report an improved mood after being outside.[15] Sit outside, even if just for a meal or a quick fifteen minutes. The sun exposure will boost your vitamin D level, and there will be lots of birds, clouds, and trees to gaze at. Many hospitals now have special outdoor sitting patios or gardens; when your doctor gives you the OK, have a loved one walk or wheel you out there.

Craft Something

Author Barbara Fredrickson suggests generating positive emotions by creating positivity portfolios.[16] A positivity portfolio is a scrapbook based around certain positive emotions that contain things you love to look at. Crafty time! If you are too ill to take a trip or get outside, flipping through a positivity portfolio will put what you value back into view.

---

14 Katherine Doheny, "Nature Has Charms That Can Reduce Stress," *Los Angeles Times* (July, 1989). *articles.latimes.com*.

15 Clare Cooper Marcus and Marni Barnes, *Healing Gardens: Therapeutic Benefits and Design Recommendations* (New York: Wiley, 1999).

16 Barbara Fredrickson, *Positivity: Groundbreaking Research Reveals How to Embrace the Hidden Strength of Positive Emotions, Overcome Negativity, and Thrive* (New York: Crown Archetype, 2009), 184–91.

You can use photos, magazine cutouts, stickers, old movie tickets, or other treasures. Visit any craft store to pick up a scrapbook of your choosing. When you feel up to it, spend an afternoon putting your positivity portfolio together. Here are a few theme ideas:

- Craft a page for each of your top ten values.

- Create a positivity portfolio around all of the things you are grateful for.

- Create a portfolio that focuses on the people you love.

- Make a vision book that details your future goals.

- Design a healing portfolio that talks about why you love your body and includes things that speak to your philosophy of healing.

- Create a bucket list portfolio of all the amazing things you have ahead of you.

- Craft a hodgepodge portfolio of everything you love.

Keep your positivity portfolio close at hand and flip through it often.

Hearing

For a long time when I was young, I used to see an osteopath for treatment. She would stretch my legs and arms in an effort to get things back into alignment. During our sessions a live pianist was in the room. It was so cool! She would play a variety of classical music, but my love for Bach's Prelude No. 1 came from that room with the sun streaming in and notes dancing off the walls. I don't remember any of the discomfort that resulted from the osteopath's exercises, but I will always have a soft spot for the slow build of that prelude. It still brings tears to my eyes.

It is easy to get swept up by a melody or lyrics that speak to your heart. This type of distraction can work wonders to move your focus toward something less needle-filled.

Take Your Soundtrack with You

While not everyone has a pianist to follow them around while they focus on their health, music is now available in a variety of electronic formats. You can download songs onto your computer and sync them with a portable MP3 player to take to the doctor's office, hospital, on a walk, out on the porch, or into any room in the house. You can get small speakers to connect to your MP3 player if headphones bug you.

Create different playlists that inspire a variety of moods. You could have one for relaxation with classical and soft instrumental music, a sentimental playlist that reminds you of when you were back in school, or a playlist of your favorite current songs. Also create a list that gives you energy, upbeat songs that prompt you to swing your hips or sing. This can be just the thing if you feel sluggish.

The online music service Spotify (*www.spotify.com*) allows you to create a variety of playlists for free on your home computer. Through Spotify and Pandora (*www .pandora.com*), another online music service, you can tailor custom "radio" stations to your liking based on a specific artist or genre of music. I sometimes forget to turn on music, but I always remember how powerful it is once I do.

Listen for Music in Nature

You can also hear music by turning to nature. Over time we have relied less and less on our hearing to predict our safety. We don't need to listen for the approaching animal to find food or to know if we're in danger, now we just have to listen for our cell phones and the ping of a new e-mail. We have become disconnected from the natural world in our daily lives. Returning to nature with our ears is one way to unplug from the stress of work, family, and that upcoming CT scan.

There are a number of ways to do this. You could open your windows, close your eyes, and listen to the wind or the birds. You can get a CD of nature sounds with waves, streams, or rain. A small indoor water fountain can put a babbling brook right in your home. It is a beautifully meditative moment to place your attention on the natural sounds around you. Connecting back with the earth is a way to reconnect with yourself.

Seek Silence

In a section on sound we have to talk about silence. Psychologist Sherry Turkle researches how technology is impacting human connection and communication. She astutely observes that we see being alone with ourselves in silence as a problem to be solved.[17] We turn on the television, tweet, update Facebook or Pinterest, text, and e-mail to solve this "problem" of being alone. We have forgotten what silence feels like. It takes practice to be truly silent, but working to be in silence and enjoy it is a beautiful gift.

Aside from cherishing silence in and of itself, there may be sounds you really want to avoid. In 2010, I came down with a really weird case of pneumonia; it didn't present itself with fever, fatigue, aches, etc., but it collapsed part of my right lung. After weeks of being out of breath, I went to the doctor's office only to be sent straight to the emergency room. They get quite concerned when they can't hear air in your lungs. I ended up needing to stay in the hospital for a few days to have a bronchoscopy and other breathing treatments to address the collapsed lung.

---

17 Sherry Turkle, "Connected, But Alone?" Video (June, 2012). *www.ted.com.*

The first room I was assigned to was a double, and the other occupant in the room had a cough that made a jet engine sound like a whisper. I felt awful for her and not so great for myself, thinking that I would be spending the night listening to her battle with severe pneumonia. Phillip ran back to our home to pick up a few things for my stay and grabbed some earplugs on his way back to the hospital. They were my lifesaver.

Sleep is the best healing modality we have. Being in a hospital or busy home can be disruptive, and cultivating silence is essential to giving our body the break it needs. Turn off the boob tube, close the windows, shut the door, put the earplugs in, and listen to nothing.

Taste

Diet is one of those things that is bound to change when you get a diagnosis. We can control our diets, and we should. Putting good stuff into our bodies is a big factor in creating health. Though diet can also be an epic brawl between your best intentions and deep-fried potato skins.

Preplan Your Meals

To make things less stressful around your sense of taste, preplan, preplan, preplan. This is the most important ingredient to eating what you say you will, and not eating what you say you won't.

Each week I make a master grocery list. On the back of the list I write down the dinners I'll be fixing during the week. On the front goes the groceries I'll need for those meals, as well as breakfast and lunch items. I take my time to create the list, grab a cookbook (or two), and go through the pantry and refrigerator and brainstorm what our meals will be. I sometimes even look over my favorite restaurant menus to think about how I could make their dishes at home. Being at the store with a list means that I don't stray toward the prebaked goodies— unless Phillip comes to the store with me. Somehow the cart always fills up quicker when he's there.

At home, I look at the back of my grocery list to determine what we're going to have for dinner. By thinking about my weekly meals once, I know that I am eating a variety of foods and getting well-balanced meals that are specific to my health.

Accommodate Special Diets

I eventually went from vegetarian to vegan—no dairy and no eggs. As I contemplated being vegan, I knew that I would miss macaroni and cheese, but I also knew that it would bloat me up like a giant Peanuts character floating down the Macy's Thanksgiving Day Parade. I'm too kind to deny myself what I'm craving; I simply figure out how to make it healthier. There are a bazillion recipe sites on the Internet, many devoted to low-fat, healthy, vegetarian or vegan cooking. Type in "healthy enchiladas recipe," "sugar-free cookies," "vegetarian lasagna," or whatever else it is your taste buds just have to have, and voilà, dinner is on the table. I did find a delicious recipe on VegNews (*www.vegnews.com*) for vegan macaroni and cheese that I make monthly. I use whole wheat pasta and add in broccoli, green beans, and zucchini for extra veggie goodness. No, they don't taste exactly the same, but some recipes are pretty darn close, and you'll feel better after you've taken the high road instead of the one that leads through the drive-through. Make sure you have lots of healthy snacks around, too. Planning takes the stress out of eating.

Recreate Your Favorite Nostalgic Foods

Another way to use your taste buds to address stress is to make some of your favorite foods from childhood. Any time I am sick, I always have to have soup and a muffin. My mom would pick them up for me at a nearby café and I associate that specific taste with feeling better. In your house is it minestrone soup? Fresh-baked bread? Casserole? Peanut butter on celery with raisins? Food can be very comforting. You may need to adjust the ingredients to create a lower calorie version, but food that brings you back to your youth is a big hug from the past.

Keeping Down Hospital Food

Now a word about hospital food. Unfortunately, in my experience medicine tends to be dragging its feet when it comes to nutrition. I once got a dietary restriction sheet that suggested I drink Kool-Aid. Seriously. If you are in the hospital, you can still manage your diet to an extent. Ask if there are any alternative menus you can choose from. Hospitals do have vegetarian, vegan, gluten-free, or other menus that you can request. Work with your nurse and/or dietician to make sure that you are comfortable with the food you are being served.

* * *

When you eat a meal, make it an event. Sit down and take the time to taste what you are eating. Savor each bite. Rediscover what food actually tastes like. You may realize that a fresh peach can make you stomp and shout with joy.

Touch

Numerous research studies have demonstrated the healing power of touch.[18] When I was in the neonatal intensive care unit, my dad observed that I needed less pain

---

18 Andrea Cooper, "The Healing Power of Touch," WebMD (2008, April). *www.webmd.com.*

medication when someone was there to stroke my leg. I even started picking up my toes for kisses. Today, I "hint" that I want my hair stroked by sneaking my hair under Phillip's hand for a bit of roll-your-eyes-back-in-your-head touch therapy.

Treat Yourself to Touch

We touch things all day long; with some thought and intention, we can make those touches aimed at relieving stress. Here are a few ways:

- Get a massage if that fits into your budget. Be sure to check with your insurance company, as some are beginning to cover this. Select hospitals also provide massage to patients if their condition would benefit from it.

- Give your pet a massage. My dogs are notorious for crowding me out on the couch; while they're there, I take advantage of pet therapy. Running my hands through their fur makes me so very happy.

- Have lots of cozy blankets around.

- Splurge on some flannel or satin sheets. Fresh sheets make the end of any day better.

- Open your windows to feel the breeze caress your skin.

- If you get chills or just like to be extra warm, hot water bottles and heating pads are a must. I've been known to take mine into the office.

- Puffy eyes, puffy anything, gets soothed with an ice pack. Frozen peas make an excellent substitute.

- When you are outside slip off your cardigan and notice how the sun's rays feel on your skin.

- If you know you are going to be recuperating for a while, get a special pair of pajamas. Ones that feel luxuriously soft. Top those off with a microfiber robe for added cushiness.

- Hold hands, cuddle, smooch, hug, and love on your loved ones.

Make Time for a Mini-facial

Is washing your face an afterthought? When the day is over, the last thing on most women's minds is taking time to cleanse, exfoliate, tone, mask, and moisturize. However, our own touch is healing as well. The ten or so minutes you spend in the bathroom getting ready for bed could be like a mini spa visit. Save that time just for yourself, no interruptions. Create a skin care routine specific to your skin type. Most involve cleansing, toning, and moisturizing. Every now and again, you can also exfoliate with a scrub or use a mask. Remove all of your makeup each evening and slowly care for your skin. It is a small way to demonstrate that you value yourself.

Smell

My favorite smell in the whole wide world is a campfire. It has this way of taking me back to a camping trip when I was nine, roasting marshmallows, dad playing the guitar, a thousand twinkling stars. Smell can quickly pull you from current stress and put you back to the place you really want to be. Think back over your life. What were some of your favorite smells? Fresh-cut grass? The sea? Mossy forest? Chocolate-chip cookies? Mom's perfume? If you have those around, that's fabulous, put the cookies in the oven. If not, you can tap into your sense of smell with aromatherapy.

Breathe in Aromatherapy

Adding essential oils to a warm bath takes a relaxing moment over the top. You can also use scented candles, incense, or a scent diffuser to fill the room with jasmine blossoms, roses, or peppermint. If you are in the hospital, a cotton ball with a few drops of your favorite essential oil is a discreet way to get the benefits of aromatherapy. Here are a few of the more popular scents and their benefits:

- Basil—eases fatigue

- Bergamot—relaxes

- Chamomile—soothes

- Eucalyptus—purifies

- Jasmine—relieves stress

- Lavender—restores balance

- Peppermint—energizes

* * *

The act of tuning in to your five senses automatically takes you out of your head, away from where stressful thoughts live. Creating an environment that leans toward peace and draws us in allows us to be distracted for a while. Your environment should nourish you. You already have enough depleting your energy without your home and your office stealing more. Look back over the suggestions for each of your senses and list a few in your journal that you will implement.

CREATING MY TEMPLE

List ways you will enhance your environment to cater to your senses and create a peaceful, nourishing space.

What to Bring to the Hospital

Sometimes the sanctuary you are creating is not in your own home. It is an unfortunate reality that many of our hospitals are too busy to operate in a way that is solely focused on healing. Hospitals have many patients, and their schedule is probably not your schedule. The lights, noise level, gadgets, and procedures can sometimes act against your body's natural healing ability.

When I was in the hospital to treat my collapsed lung, the nurse gave me a Pepcid, a medication used to help treat stomach ulcers by reducing acid levels. She said research has shown that just being in the hospital is stressful enough to give a patient an ulcer. They began giving all patients Pepcid to guard against the physical impact of hospital stress. Not surprising, since my 4:00 A.M. wake-up call was always jarring fluorescent lights and a needle stick.

Do not assume that the hospital will have everything you want. If you have some advance notice, say, a surgery coming up, you can pack a bag of the things that will help you feel more comfortable. If you go in for an emergency, once things have calmed you can send a friend or a family member back to pack your bag.

Here is an exhaustive list of everything you might need or want for your hospital stay:

- Identification

- Insurance card

- Medical record number or health center card

- List of your medications with doses and when you last took them, including any over-the-counter medications you take

- The name and phone number of your primary care physician or other specialists

- Any records, X-rays, or test results you have that the hospital may not have

- Documents that require your doctor's signature—for workers' comp, work absence, disability, etc.

- Advanced health care directive (a.k.a. a living will)—bring a copy if you have one prepared, or the hospital can assist you with this

- An address book with phone numbers and e-mail addresses of important people who should be notified when your surgery is a success

- Pillow if you prefer your own

- Warm plush blanket

- Photo album of the people you love or small framed pictures

- Comforting symbol of your faith

- Your positivity portfolio

- MP3 player with your favorite music

- Magazines

- Books or an e-reader

- Funny or relaxing DVDs (check to see if your hospital has a player)

- Puzzle, Sudoku, or crossword books

- Journal

- Pen and paper

- Laptop

- Essential oil for a cotton ball

- Favorite *healthy* snack foods if you are not on a restricted diet

- Earplugs

- Sleeping mask

- Toothbrush and toothpaste

- A change or two of comfortable, very loose clothing

- Slippers

- Tennis shoes

- Socks and underwear, several pairs of each

- Cozy bathrobe

- Lip balm

- Hairbrush and hair ties (I find it easiest to keep my hair in a low ponytail or French braid while in the hospital.)

- A favorite yummy body lotion

- Razors and makeup if you are daring

- Glasses and/or contacts with appropriate storage and solution

- Other personal items: hearing aids, braces, etc.

Do not bring any jewelry or valuables with you to the hospital. You won't be able to wear the jewelry, and you don't want to have to worry about the valuables. You may want to have a list of what you'd want for a hospital stay ready in case you need to be admitted unexpectedly.

Hospitals are not the most fun place on the planet, but they can be made into your own personal healing temple away from home. Our dog Abbey didn't want to be in her cage for five weeks, but she knew it was the best place for her at the time.

A Conversation with Kelly Young, Rheumatoid Arthritis Crusader

Kelly Young is a 2011 WebMD Health Hero, a member of the Mayo Clinic Center for Social Media Advisory Board, a crusading rheumatoid arthritis (RA) advocate, and a minister's wife and mother of five. Visit her at: *www.rawarrior.com.*

"I've lived most of my life as a very healthy, strong person. [I am] very self-reliant and [spent] a lot of time and effort taking care of others. When I give a talk, I like to show a picture of myself on my ladder. One summer, I spread two tons of concrete stucco on the outside of my house. I did a lot of things like that because I thought they needed to be done."

After Kelly gave birth to her fifth child, she had a "very sudden onset of permanent inflammation" that affected all of her joints. She explained that RA can manifest differently in different people. "Some people are like lupus patients and they flare a few times a year. Some people are well and sometimes even have remissions, but there is a pretty good-sized portion of people like me who actually don't flare, they just have constant inflammation. It's just varying which joints are worse or whether their eyes are worse or their lungs are." She has been managing the constant inflammation of RA for six years. After trying six different treatments in those six years, Kelly began to discover other people with RA who were looking for answers. That's when she felt called to become an advocate.

Because RA impacts her life in such an encompassing way, Kelly has had to adjust her environment and activity level to cater to her body's new requirements. "I went from being able to go to the beach and run for an hour or two, play tennis with my kids, and do lots of other things, to not being able to wash dishes. I can't walk very far; it hurts to walk at all. I start walking, and within a few minutes I'm slowing down, and then I'm really dragging myself. Within a few more minutes it's very, very difficult because my knees, my hips, all my toes, my ankles, they're all in a flare and everything is kind of screaming in flare. I do get to a point where I can't move at all. It's really hard. It's a really hard way to live, so I make a lot of choices about what I can't do and can do."

One of the challenges with RA, as with many other chronic illnesses, is that symptoms are not readily visible. It can be difficult to explain to others that you are unable to do something when you look healthy. For Kelly, this challenge came down to finding balance in what she expects from her body. "You not only have to be gracious enough with others and yourself to say where those limits are, but you have to be able to admit that you need to adjust your limits and say, 'Today I can't do this, I can only do that.'"

I asked Kelly how that graciousness extended to her environment, her house, and the places she visits. Her answer started with the place she was sitting while we talked. "I have this chair that I love. It was actually a chair I got at the Salvation Army for ten dollars, but I had this fabric that was really beautiful and soft. I created a new cushion, pillows, and fringe for the chair, so it's really soft. I have pillows even for my elbows and a special stool, so I'm really comfortable because I need to have my knees supported. I've constructed an environment that I can manage at home."

The challenges of traveling with RA leave a lot of people homebound. Kelly was surprised to discover that she was living close to a few fellow patients. "It's really hard to travel because as soon as you go anywhere else, you're looking around, and there's not a chair that's just right, or a place where you can straighten your knees and at the same time shift the weight off your hips for a minute. I didn't know until after I started writing my blog that there were a couple of women here in my neighborhood [with RA] that found me online, on Facebook, and they were right here!"

Because Kelly's advocacy work and social network requires her to travel from time to time she has come up with a list of things that are must-brings when she's away from home. This starts with her mode of transportation. "I have my truck, my Suburban. It has really nice big leather seats with lots of electric buttons to adjust them. It's really important to be comfortable, even going to a friend's house. If I'm going to be gone from my house for a few hours, I have a small travel pillow, and I have a throw, and I have a big pillow. My shoes are not going to be on my feet unless they absolutely have to be, and I have socks in case my feet get cold in that environment. I have this little case full of tons of different prescription medicines and a list of what the medicines are and when the last time I took them is. That's with me wherever I am. I always have a water bottle, and I almost always have a little cracker package or some bit of food in case I need to take medication. I just bring all that with me everywhere I go."

Kelly got sick just as she was starting to decorate the house she lives in now, but her family stepped in to provide conveniences that ease the stress on Kelly's joints. "My kids have bought me so many things. They bought me a little lap desk to put my laptop on, so I don't have the weight of it on my hips. It (the desk) can adjust depending on what my position is. I talk on the phone a lot, so we've gotten a headset for the phone, and we just got a new radio with big easy buttons on it because the old radio that I had in my room was actually a dial that I had to turn instead of buttons that you push and hold down."

One key to retaining independence for Kelly centers around how much an object weighs. "We're always looking for things that are not heavy. Before there is even bone damage, or anything you can see on an X-ray, there's an immediate weakening of the tendon. So you could pick up something like a milk jug or an iron, which would be fine one day, and then the very next day, if you have a joint affected, you can't pick it up the way you could before. I've pretty much replaced everything, whether it's the hair dryer, hairbrush, or anything I can think of. When I buy a purse, a bag, a laptop, camera, anything I want, it's all about picking them up and researching and find out what's the lightest one that would be comfortable so that I can still do that [activity]."

For some patients, their RA symptoms vary from day to day and year to year, but Kelly's RA has been a daily marathon of inflammation. I asked her how she copes with, as she describes it, the "drudgery" of knowing that every day is the same. Her insight was touching. "You become a more optimistic person that's more outward focused. The whole focus of your life can't be yourself and your abilities, and 'look at me, and what I can do.' I really delight in watching my kids. I couldn't play tennis anymore, but I would go to the tennis matches and I would watch them play tennis. I would be thrilled to watch them do whatever they can do. You become more outward focused and less selfish, less self-focused. I've seen that in so many people.

"I tend to think that it's living with a chronic illness that starts to bring that out in people because I've seen so many people with RA who have such a beautiful spirit. They're so generous. They lift other people up and always try to be positive, think for the best, and be optimistic even though they go through one treatment after another because the disease is progressive. You kind of know that next year you probably won't be better than this year, it'll be the same or a little worse. There are grief stages that you go through in the beginning, but then once it becomes chronic and it's long-term and you've reasoned with it, you pass over into a more accepting, mature outlook toward life—where it is, what it is—and you just live. You try to look outward and focus on others." Kelly jokes with me that it is "almost like an enforced spiritual maturity, where you would hope people would get there in their life eventually anyway, but it forces you to get there sooner."

Kelly's life with five kids and living with RA have helped her evolve into a low-stress person. She has had to learn a great deal about flexibility and acceptance. When she does face a tough situation, she practices her own advice. "Last night I had to do this shot, and it makes me nauseous for a couple of days. I don't want the medicine. I don't want to do it. I have to force myself to do it."

> [Illness is] almost like an enforced spiritual maturity, where you would hope people would get there in their life eventually anyway, but it forces you to get there sooner.

She took to Twitter and posted, "'I have to go pay some bills now and then do that shot that makes me sick to my stomach for two days, so what's going to be my reward?' I have told people so many times, 'reward yourself.' And then I got a whole bunch of people responding to me [with recommendations]: 'Oh, go get a Coke Slurpee. That's so good for nausea.' 'Oh, buy yourself a dress, you so much deserve it.' A whole bunch of different ideas. We went and picked up sushi. We got fresh ginger with it. Did you know ginger fights nausea? On top of thinking it was wonderful to go and get some sushi because it was a treat, we knew that I could say, 'this is the ginger that's going to cure the nausea, so I'm going to feel a lot better tomorrow.'" She says she feels guilty for using food as a reward because occasionally the reward is ice cream, but I too have been known to snag a cupcake after a particularly hard doctor appointment or test. Sometimes whatever gets you through is the thing to do.

RA has shifted Kelly's life 180 degrees. I asked how that has impacted her perception of life. Her answer demonstrates the honest bravery that comes with the time and maturity of coping with a chronic illness. "I used to think I could do anything, it would just take me longer than others. My mom used to say 'you're a bull and just charge into life.' That really gets adjusted by RA. It's a really big attitude adjustment. You can't control everything. You can't fix everything. You can't just do everything. But you can still find your way through."

Kelly continues to inspire others on her blog and popular Facebook page by sharing the realities and lessons RA teaches her every day.

HEALTH TIPS

- Your immune system needs all the energy it can get. Your environment should add to that energy, not drain it.

- Choose one or two personal retreats in your home or office that provide rest and relaxation.

- Use your five senses to create a peaceful space.

- Plan, organize, and get help from friends and family to make creating and maintaining a personal sanctuary easier.

- Have a list of what you would want for a hospital stay ready. The hospital can be a place of calm healing with some personal touches.

CHAPTER 6

Call in the Troops and Put Them Through Boot Camp

The Bay Bridge spans 8.4 miles to connect Oakland with San Francisco. In 1989, a 7.1-magnitude earthquake rocked the entire Bay Area. During the quake, a 250-ton piece of the Bay Bridge's upper deck collapsed. Even though the bridge was repaired, and remarkably opened a month after the quake, engineers were left to ponder how to strengthen the bridge to withstand future quakes and protect the 280,000 cars that carry commuters, visitors, and families with little ones tucked into car seats across the bridge each day.[19]

The California Department of Transportation realized that they needed a new bridge. Building the original Bay Bridge in 1936 was no easy feat, and now they are doing it again, this time with a state-of-the-art support system. As you drive into the city, you can see the new bridge mirroring the dips and supports of the original.

Life is the Bay Bridge, and illness is the 7.1-magnitude earthquake. Without support, the stress of a quake can collapse what may seem to be concrete-tough. The people you surround yourself with are the reinforced steel that allow the bridge to sway with earthquakes while keeping everything intact.

---

19 "Bay Bridge Construction Corridor Overview," The San Francisco-Oakland Bay Bridge Seismic Safety Projects, (2012). *baybridgeinfo.org.*

What's the Big Deal About Support?

A while back I asked my mom "How did you make it through the first few years after I was born with all that was going on?" Her answer, "I had so much support. Your dad was there, and we had a lot of family and friends helping. Your doctors were also absolutely wonderful. It allowed me to completely focus on your healing." That is what support does. It enables you to put your full attention on healing.

Humans are social animals. It is built into our DNA. Since the time we were hunting, gathering, and living in caves, we have needed each other to survive. Study after study has shown that strong social ties are one of the best predictors of happiness, longevity, and health.[20]

The irony is that when you don't feel well, you don't feel like being a social butterfly. Relationships take time and energy, something that is at a premium when you're healing. You may also assume that reaching out to others while you're sick is burdening them with your challenges. This can burden *you* with the pressure to be positive.

After Barbara Ehrenreich, author of *Bright-Sided*, was diagnosed with breast cancer, she turned to an online breast cancer forum to seek support and read about the journeys of other women facing her diagnosis. What she found was a community stubbornly committed to seeing breast cancer in a positive light. There is absolutely nothing wrong with turning lemons into lemonade; however, room needs to be allowed for the natural emotions of fear, anger, and frustration that tag along with a diagnosis like cancer. When Ehrenreich posted a comment about her honest emotions, she was met with reprimand

---

20 *Today's Research on Aging*, (June 2009), Population Reference Bureau, No. 17.

and urges to see a counselor immediately.[21] Though it has been disproved, there is widespread belief that our very survival depends on being optimistic.[22] This may compel a woman to only share positive thoughts with others. Wanting to be strong, resilient, and an example of grace can lead to a denial of our natural emotions with others, and even with ourselves.

One of the hardest things I have had to do is tell my mom that it was time to be listed for a kidney transplant. I knew I was breaking her heart. She was strong on the phone, and I cushioned the news with lots of statements like "I'm fine. Everything will be OK. I have no doubt that we will find a good donor. I feel well now." I didn't share the tough stuff. I didn't tell her that I was scared, worried, and disappointed with my body. I wanted to minimize her pain by hiding my own. In fact, many of the conversations I had went like that. I didn't want people to worry about me. I became so good at my "bad news" speech, I even convinced myself that I was OK with this turn of events. I wanted to be positive.

After going through the transplant testing, I started to realized that "I'm fine" wasn't really true. What I was trying to make a small deal was a big deal, a life-changing deal. I had been giving all of the support and hadn't asked for any of my own. I needed support. I needed a friend. Not someone to fix it, or to help me be positive, but someone to listen and to let me know that it was OK to feel how I was feeling.

Illness is inherently vulnerable. Sharing the pain, frustration, and sadness with your loved ones can be

---

21 Barbara Ehrenreich, *Bright-Sided: How the Relentless Promotion of Positive Thinking Has Undermined America* (New York: Metropolitan Books, 2009), 34–35.

22 Richard Sloan, "A Fighting Spirit Won't Save Your Life," *The New York Times* (January, 2009). *www.nytimes.com*.

intimidating, but it can be beneficial too. Having someone witness your experience, in all its messiness, can help you find meaning. It is extremely validating to have someone hear what you are going through. It is not only the positive stuff we need to share with others—it is the whole of the human experience. Connecting in honesty is liberating for both the patient and their supporter.

That said, having support is not only about having a shoulder to wipe your snotty tears on. Support does not have to be that heavy all the time. There are a host of reasons to seek out others:

- Needing to laugh

- Wanting to be distracted

- Wanting to talk about last night's episode of *American Idol*

- Needing a hug

- Not wanting to go to the doctor alone

- Needing help with chores, cooking, changing bandages, mobility, picking up the kids, or picking the right outfit

- Wanting a reminder that everything is going to be OK

- Longing for confirmation that you are beautiful with the bedhead and splotchy completion

- Wanting a bucket list buddy for your adventures

- Celebrating health victories with someone by jumping up and down in squeaky excitement

- Needing a point of contact for extended friends and family

- Getting caught up on the office gossip

- Wanting to discuss the meaning of life

- Needing a confidant who knows your goals and can make decisions if you are unable to

- Wanting a mom, someone to make you soup, tuck you in, and kiss your forehead

Let people in whichever way you are comfortable with. If you take the risk to share the tough with the good, I know you'll be amazed at how deep your relationships become.

Who Will Support You?

When you're choosing your support team, it is helpful to start with who *isn't* a good candidate. Not everyone you are already close with will be able to provide the type of support you need. People tend to show their true colors when the you-know-what hits the fan, and some of your relationships may not withstand the additional weight of illness. We all have our own beliefs and baggage following us around in life. For some, facing illness triggers painful memories or fears of their own. You are not responsible for other people's reactions. Their stuff is their stuff. Hurtful, insensitive, or ignorant comments are not about you. Coping with illness is foreign territory for many, and they have not yet figured out what is appropriate and what is just plain wrong. Do not feel guilty for distancing yourself from people who drain your energy and make you feel more stressed.

Some common energy-drainers include:

- "The Unwelcome Advice-Giver"—This is someone who feels the need to share his opinion on everything about your treatment. He tells you to take this herb or to see his chiropractor all without your asking. His intentions are in the right place, but it can be exhausting to continually defend the approach you take with your health.

- "The Dictator"—This is the Unwelcome Advice-Giver to the extreme. Someone like this absolutely insist that you do things her way and will turn on you if you don't.

- "The Overtalker"—I am all for listening, but this person is just talking to hear the sound of her own voice. If you do get a word in edgewise, the conversation is quickly turned back to her and how her aunt had the exact same thing as you. She will continue for another forty-five minutes describing the horrific side effects of the medicine you just started taking and can look forward to. This relationship is all give.

- "The Denier"—This is someone who refuses to accept that you're ill. He says that illness is all in the mind or that you're making a bigger deal out of your condition than it is. Conversations with the Denier make you question your very sanity.

- "The Critic"—This "supporter" continually puts you down with the guise of "just trying to help." She is critical of your choices and seems to feel that you are directly responsible for your illness.

Anyone who requires more energy than you get in return is not a candidate to join your support team. This doesn't mean that things can't change with a few heartfelt conversations. Some people may truly want to be on your team, but they just don't know how. However, if talking it out doesn't change anything, give yourself a break and look elsewhere for support.

Your support system may be obvious. Phillip will be there to listen to the doctor's instructions and help me to the bathroom after surgery. He'll hold me tight, pick up prescriptions, tell me when I'm being too dramatic, and surprise me with magazines and my favorite soup. He is my foundation. But if your support team consists of only one person, you have built a table with only one leg, and you won't be able to balance for long. Caregivers are also coping with the stress of your illness and need breaks from time to time. Having multiple people you can turn to is adding the second, third, and fourth legs to your table.

Most people have natural instincts to support others in loving and generous ways. It is not hard to find people who genuinely want to reach out in compassion. When thinking about who you want to include in your team, consider adding people with these qualities:

- They are empathetic. They are able to be present with your pain.

- They do not take on your pain. They allow you to feel what you are feeling without becoming emotionally overwhelmed themselves.

- They listen without directing the conversation or attempting to change how you experience your illness.

- They help you stay focused on the things you can control.

- They are honest with you even when you don't want to hear it.

- They respect your boundaries and your requests.

- They accept what you are going through without trying to fix or condemn it.

There are a number of people who will fit the above description. You can look to your immediate family, extended family, friends, church, co-workers, health care providers, therapist, spiritual advisor, or support group. On the Internet you can find a support forum for every major and obscure illness out there. Many illnesses have national conferences where you can meet other patients and hear the latest in stem cells and treatment options. I know people who have met lifelong friends through such conferences.

It is up to you to decide how public to make your health. For some, posting updates on Facebook about doctor appointments or the new rash that just showed up feels comforting, but for others it is too exposing.

Grab your journal and write down your list of supporters. Think about who you'd call when you need the exact person that will meet you for coffee and take your mind off your illness, when you got a bad test result and need to vent, or when you're overwhelmed with paperwork. People want to be there for you. They just need to be asked and told how they can best support you.

YOUR SUPPORT TEAM

Create a list of the people and professionals who support your health and healing.

Calling in the Professionals

In June of 2011, the phone rang and I picked it up to hear a voice I hadn't heard in twenty-four years. It was Dr. Hardy Hendren.

When I was eighteen months old, I needed an exotic reconstruction to reverse a colostomy created shortly after I was born. My doctors at San Diego Children's Hospital were not yet experienced in this area, and they presented my parents with a decision: they could attempt (not a great word) the surgery at San Diego Children's, or we could all fly to Boston for five weeks to have the expert and originator of this surgery perform it. That expert was Dr. Hardy Hendren.

Dr. Hendren's colleagues in Boston call him "Hardly Human" because he can operate for twenty-four hours straight.[23] He has devoted his life to his family and to perfecting complex gastrointestinal and urologic surgeries. My parents jumped at the chance to have the magician work his magic.

I had two successful surgeries during our stay in Boston. Over the years, each time Dr. Hendren visited Southern California, he would make a point of following up with my family. Now here he was on the phone wanting to know how I was doing. He was concerned about my kidney and gave me a list of things to check on with my doctors. He remembered my family and said that he still had a thank-you note from my mom. In his eighties and continuing to work part-time, Dr. Hendren was searching out the two hundred–plus patients he had performed similar surgeries on to see how they were doing now. His concern and dedication was a warm cashmere blanket on a frosty morning.

There are amazing healers out there, professionals who have profound concern for their patients' well-being. For each doctor who has poor bedside manner, each technician who is rushed, each therapist who doesn't understand, there are a multitude of compassionate and talented people who have a goal of helping you heal. These people are on your support team as well.

---

23 G. Wayne Miller, *The Work of Human Hands* (New York: Random House, 1993), 29–30.

In the overwhelm and confusion of illness, it is common for women to lose their voice. You get to decide who participates in your care. If you are unhappy with the level of care you receive, ask for a second opinion and seek out a better fit. It is vital that you trust the professionals on your support team. You need to be comfortable with their values, their ability to listen, and their credentials.

The most obvious members of your professional team are doctors, but you can find professionals to support you in a variety of areas.

- Doctor—Your doctor must be well trained in the area of your illness, including appropriate board certifications. It is also important that he listen to you with his full attention. Trust is fundamental. If you don't trust your doctor, you will be less inclined to follow his recommendations.

- Therapist—If you feel emotionally overwhelmed or are concerned that you are stuck in stress and worry, do not hesitate to plant yourself on someone's couch with some tissues. A therapist is talented at helping you process the massive changes in your life. She can help you grieve the loss of the life you knew and accept the reality that you are in. A therapist is good listeners by nature and can be helpful if you are uncomfortable talking about your emotions with friends or family.

- Life Coach and/or Health Coach—If your care involves lifestyle changes, a coach can help you determine appropriate goals, design an action plan, and get you past obstacles. Coaches are trained listeners, motivators, and action-oriented professionals who will keep you on track.

- Trainer and/or Nutritionist—Personal trainers and nutritionists are skilled at teaching you about your body and what it needs. They can design a workout or food plan specific to your health concerns. They will also help keep you accountable.

- Religious/Spiritual Leader—Health often brings up issues of faith. When we lose control in life, many times we turn upward or inward to discover strength in a power greater than our own. Religious or spiritual leaders are skilled at assisting you with your journey and counseling you on questions of faith.

- Naturopath/Chiropractor/Acupuncturist/Massage Therapist—Alternative therapies are gaining in popularity as people seek the wisdom of ancient healing traditions. Many insurance companies are beginning to recognize the benefits of these therapies and now cover select services. If you feel that you want to explore options outside of traditional medicine, be sure to fully investigate the practitioner you choose to work with. You need to trust her and her credentials just as much as you would a doctor's.

When you are assembling your professional team, pay attention to how supported you feel by them. You can hire, fire, and give feedback to the professionals you work with. Just as with your personal relationships, your professional relationships should not take more energy than they give.

To find the best providers in your area, ask for referrals from friends, family, co-workers, and health care providers you are already working with. Many professionals maintain websites where they post articles or a blog where you can learn about their work and philosophy around healing. This will help with prescreening who you want to meet face-to-face. When you meet with a new professional, bring a list of questions that address your health concerns and the level of care you expect. Some questions may include:

- How long have you been practicing?

- How many cases have you handled similar to mine?

- What training have you received? Are you board certified? In what specialties?

- What is your typical course of treatment when addressing my condition?

- How long will our appointments last? (The national average is a measly eighteen minutes.[24])

- What results do you expect from working together?

- On average, how long does it take to achieve results?

- What is your approach to care?

- What motivates you?

- Do you support alternative treatments?

- How long does it take your office to return e-mails and phone calls?

From your initial conversation, you will have a sense about whether you want this person to know intimate details about your bathroom habits or not. If you don't feel comfortable there is no shame in thanking them for their time and moving on.

---

24 Brenda Goodman, "The 18-minute Doctor's Appointment Challenge," *Arthritis Today, www.arthritistoday.org.*

If you notice that you are bouncing from one doctor to the next and never finding a good fit, it may be less about the health care provider and more about the diagnosis and treatment you are facing. The fear of a diagnosis can send you endlessly in search of someone to tell you what you want to hear instead of what the reality is. Ask yourself if your third, fourth, and fifth opinions were obtained out of fear. If so, therapists are great at working through fear so that you can get on with treatment.

When you are surrounded by people you trust, you are able to place your attention on healing instead of second-guessing your health care provider.

Financial Support

At some point we've got to talk about finances. It is one of the biggest stresses families face when coping with illness, and it is an area where support becomes essential.

Traveling to Boston for five weeks to have a reconstructive surgery is not cheap. My father was a self-employed painting contractor, and my mother did not return to work after I was born because of the extensive care I required. We did not have health insurance. Medi-Cal and California Children's Services funded the majority of my surgeries and care, but getting to Boston was a big hurdle. My parents were unwilling to compromise on my care and needed to find a way to get all of us across the country to see Dr. Hendren. We needed to ask for help.

> Asking for financial help is never easy. It requires you to put your health above your ego and get creative.

Asking for financial help is never easy. It requires you to put your health above your ego and get creative. My dad knew how much our plane tickets would cost and began writing letters. He wrote to a variety of companies that participated in charitable giving and asked if they would sponsor our trip to Boston. One company did. My parents kept them updated on my progress and they paid for us to get where we needed to be.

Managing your finances with illness means that you will have increased health expenses from doctor visits, co-pays, deductibles, prescriptions, and additional healing therapies. Many times those increases are coupled with decreased income if you need to take unpaid time off, go on disability, leave the workforce, or switch to a lower stress, and potentially lower paying, job. The conflicting forces of increased expenses and decreased income can do a number on your bank account and stress level.

Does talking about money make you want to hide under the covers? Ignoring your finances only makes financial stress worse in the long run. Facing it and putting a plan in place will help you feel more relaxed and empowered. If you need help, grab your spouse, a trusted friend, or a financial professional to help you.

The first thing to do is get organized. You need to know what your *current* household income and expenses are. There are a number of computer software programs as well as online systems to help you with this. I am a fan of Mint (*www.mint.com*). It is a secure and easy-to-use financial management tool. If you use online banking, you can download all of your transactions to your financial management program and track your bills, spending, budget, and financial goals all automatically, which saves time and energy. Most programs have tutorials in their help sections which will assist with learning the ins and outs of your new finance tool. This is electronic support at its best.

Once you've got everything set up, look at what your monthly household income and expenses are. Is there a gap? Do you spend more than you earn? If so, there are two things you can do to bridge the gap: decrease your expenses and/or increase your income.

Tackle your expenses first. Divide your expenses into two categories: "must" and "would be nice." Your "musts" are your rent, groceries, utilities—the things you need to survive. Your "would be nice" expenses are clothing, restaurants, gym membership, cable (yes, cable)—the things you want. Go back over your "must" list and move anything that is not absolutely essential for your survival over to the "would be nice" side. For instance, is a second family car a must? With your family, think of unique ways that you can cut back on your spending.

Now compare your list of "musts" with your income. Is there still a gap? If so, there are a number of government programs and other resources available to assist people who are dealing with illness. I have put together a list in Appendix B for your reference.

There are so many programs and services available it can be overwhelming to determine which ones you qualify for. No need to stress. Seek out support. The first place to look would be your hospital social worker, case manager, or patient advocate. Many hospitals also have financial counseling services available. You simply need to begin asking and people in your health network will point you in the right direction. These professionals will be able to help you understand what benefits and services may be available to you as well as help you set up a payment plan for existing medical bills.

If you are employed, your company's human resources representative is another person to see. She can help you understand your sick time allocation, potential disability benefits, and health insurance benefits. Sometimes employees come together to donate sick or vacation time to a co-worker who is coping with a prolonged illness so that they do not lose income. If this is a possibility at your company, human resources would be the department to set this up. Keep in mind that the Family and Medical Leave Act states that if you have worked more than one year in a company with more than fifty employees you are entitled to twelve weeks of unpaid leave. You would need to disclose your health status and the reason for your leave, but you would be guaranteed a job upon your return.

Also consider bridging the gap between your income and expenses by exploring unusual means for generating funds, just as my dad did when he found a company to purchase our plane tickets to Boston. Civic organizations, charitable foundations, health associations, community groups, and religious organizations are all places to look for assistance. Asking is not easy, but your health needs you to put discomfort aside and be a bit vulnerable to receive the support of others. In this digital age we live in, you can even set up online donations. Give-Forward (*www.giveforward.com*) allows you to create a web page to receive credit card or PayPal donations from concerned friends and family.

Lastly, be sure to look at your existing medical benefits. An unexpected hospital stay can add up quickly if your annual premium is high. After I got on the transplant list, during the next open enrollment Phillip and I switched from a PPO health insurance plan to an HMO. While the PPO would allow us to see specialty providers without a referral, it also had higher co-pays and annual premiums. After having seen our medical expenses creep up the year prior, we forwent the luxury of plan flexibility for additional financial benefits given the large expense that is in our future.

There are expenses you can cut and there are funds you can find. You will need to get clear about what you need and speak up to ask for it. I know you will be surprised by the financial support that is available.

Communicating with Your Support Team

Sixteen of us were huddled in a classroom, here to learn about the ins and outs of receiving a kidney transplant. I glanced around the room. We all looked nervous. I also noticed that I didn't fit the profile of someone who should be in this class. I am young and haven't yet needed dialysis. I wanted to stand up, grab my purse, and say "I'm sorry, I think I've made a mistake. I must be in the wrong room. I don't really need a transplant," while backing slowly toward the door. But I sat, like a good patient, in silence as the nurse explained that kidney cells don't regenerate like other cells in the body do. Once they are gone, they are gone. The only current treatments for kidney failure are transplant or dialysis.

After the class was over, Phillip and I were back in the lobby waiting to see the doctor for my physical exam. I said, "I don't belong here." Phillip responded by saying, "OK, what do we do about that?" I know he desperately wants to fix this for me. He doesn't want me to be in pain. He wants my body to be as healthy as I picture myself to be.

It is in our nature to want to fix things. It is the spirit of the industrial revolution. The entrepreneur in us pushes against the way things are until a solution pops out. The issue is that sometimes the solution is not yet available, or the solution does not exist, or the solution does not apply, or the solution is too sucky to pursue. Often we need our supporters to accept us and our illness as is without trying to fix what's wrong.

I answered my husband's question by saying, "We don't do anything. We sit and wait to see the doctor" as I moved my hand over to nestle in his. The goal for communicating with your support team is to invite them to support you in the ways that you need.

Do Your Part First

Even though you have a lot on your plate right now, relationships are still a two-way street. You might need to be the one to reach out first. You may be feeling isolated, but no one will know that unless you make the decision to un-isolate yourself. Your friends and family have full and busy lives too, even though they care for you and want to support you. If you need support, be the one to pick up the phone. Sometimes people just don't know what to say or how to help, so you will need to guide them through this new territory.

It is a rare gift to really be listened to. You may have a lot to update your supporters on with test results or the new treatment you've tried, but take a moment to hear what's going on in your supporter's life. You may not have the energy to be the active friend you used to be, but you can still listen.

The human body is fascinating, and we want to share our new knowledge and connect through the intimate details of how nauseated we are or how we now have restless legs syndrome. For some people, it is too much. Be mindful of when you may be oversharing by listening to your supporter's response. It takes energy to listen to the rough edges that life has, and your supporter may have reached his or her limit. If you feel they have tuned out or are overwhelmed, dial it back and change the subject to the latest episode of *Modern Family*. Listening in this way demonstrates that you value your supporter.

Forgiveness is also something you'll need to become familiar with. Not everyone knows the Hallmark thing to say, or that you've already tried acupuncture, or that you are aware of the side effect of your recent prescription, or that you don't want to hear about their second cousin who died from what you've got. If you hear rude, insensitive, or ignorant comments, gracefully say thank you and change the subject. If you're feeling particularly snarky, you can say, "I appreciate your sharing, but I am comfortable with my diagnosis and treatment." Forgive and move on.

> If you hear rude, insensitive, or ignorant comments, gracefully say thank you and change the subject.

Communicating Bad News

A diagnosis can be just as hard on your loved ones as it is on you. It is our spouse's and parents' job to protect us. It is our children's job to see us as invincible. It is our friends' job to know that we can overcome anything. Your news is messing with their job descriptions. Getting diagnosed is a helpless feeling for all involved. You are being asked to put your trust into the medical community and lean on faith to walk into the unknown. It is never easy to deliver bad news, but there are a few ways to help yourself and the people around you support each other.

- Start by sharing the facts as you understand them. Answer questions to the best of your ability.

- Always be honest. People will feel hurt if things are different than you originally communicated. Believe that people can cope with and accept the truth. Even with younger children, be honest in age appropriate ways.

- Don't apologize. Your family and friends know that you didn't choose your illness.

- Be authentic. This is how you connect with others. There is no need to sugarcoat it or to "be the strong one."

- Understand that this is a loss for them too. Allow your friends and family to grieve with you. Your relationships may need to change, at least temporarily, and they will be making adjustments also.

- Allow others to have their own reaction. You may hear responses of denial, confusion, anger, or frustration. These emotional states will pass.

Ask for What You Need

This is hard for us women. We are givers. However, other people are not mind readers. People love and support us in the way *they* would want to be supported, not necessarily in the ways that we need support.

Before each of my kidney checkups, I have blood work done so that the doctor and I have something to review. I had an appointment coming up early Friday morning and went in on Thursday at 8:00 A.M. to do the blood work. Early Thursday afternoon, the doctor called. My labs had gotten worse and he needed to adjust one of my medications. I thought, is it so bad he couldn't wait until tomorrow morning to make the adjustment? During our call, he also asked where I was at in the transplant process and seemed glad to know that we were moving through the testing. I ended our call wholly deflated.

That night in bed, I told Phillip that I was scared. My darling husband tried to calm my fears and help me accept what was going on. That wasn't what I needed at the moment. I told Phillip that I just wanted to feel sad and cry. He put his arm around me and I buried my head in his chest. Perfect.

When you speak up and say what you need, the person you're asking for help feels useful. It is frustrating to provide help that isn't welcome. Avoid confusion and just say what it is that you need. "I need someone to listen. I need to cry. I need prayers. I need to be alone for awhile. I need an advocate at the doctor. I need visitors. I need sleep. I need a road trip. I need help with the dishes. I need help with the finances. I need naughty time!" Direct requests made with appreciation are invaluable.

Set Boundaries

Setting boundaries is another type of asking for what we need. Just as people support you in the way they would want to be supported, they also assume your boundaries are the same as their boundaries. When friends, family, co-workers, or even strangers make you feel uncomfortable, it is time to set a boundary. Be clear, concise, and firm. If something is too much for you, if you don't wish to share the details of your treatment, or if you need to rest, say so.

Communicate Through Writing

If you don't feel comfortable delivering bad news, asking for what you need, or setting boundaries in person, there is no harm in sending a letter. With e-mail, the news can travel as fast as you want to send it. This also gives those who you're communicating with time to process your request and prepare their response.

There are a number of ways to communicate news about your health on a larger scale, which saves you the time and energy of contacting people one by one.

- Start a blog. Many hospitals are now beginning to offer individual web pages for patients. Caring-Bridge (*www.caringbridge.com*) is a nonprofit that connects patients with their loved ones through individual blogs. You can change the privacy settings to enable only close friends and family to view your updates.

- Create an e-mail distribution list. Gather the e-mail addresses of people who will want updates and group them together with a distribution list. Most e-mail servers have distribution list capabilities. You, or a representative for you, can write and send updates after milestones are reached in your care.

- Post updates on Facebook. If you are comfortable sharing your illness publicly, you can use Facebook as a quick way to reach the people you know.

One of the most common things to come out of illness is the realization of how important our loved ones are. Asking for support is an act of vulnerability that may feel awkward, but it is what helps us connect with the people we love most.

A Conversation with Nicole Lemelle, Inspired Blogger and Activist with Multiple Sclerosis

Nicole Lemelle is living fully with secondary progressive Multiple Sclerosis (MS). She is a blogger and activist who

inspires others by sharing her journey. Visit her at: *www
.mynewnormals.com.*

"For so long, I was so mad. The first nine years of
my diagnosis I was able to do everything normal, fine. I
knew I had MS, but it didn't really stop me from doing
anything I wanted to do. I probably took that for granted.

"Once MS came out of the closet and other people
could see it, it started dictating my life. It took away so
much. I just was so angry about it because it changed the
geography of my life. I could no longer live in Maryland,
I could no longer drive, I could no longer work. I had to
accept those things. It's an ongoing process; I have to
accept it again, and again, and again because it's always
changing."

Nicole Lemelle was diagnosed with MS during her
senior year of college. For the first nine years, her MS
was relatively stable. As she says, "I only had symptoms
that were known to me." Over the last three years, however, her MS has progressed. "I had trouble walking. I
couldn't drive anymore, and I couldn't work anymore."
This was the point that support became essential to
Nicole's management of her illness.

Though MS has limited Nicole's mobility and increased
her fatigue, her husband recognizes the abilities she still
has and nudges her to keep them. "I get out and do a lot of
things thanks to my husband. He's a very good caregiver.
He is probably the foundation to why I'm able to do as
much as I do, because when I don't feel like it, he kind of
pushes me outside."

I asked Nicole how her relationship with her husband
has had to adjust. Her answer beams with self-awareness.
"I think that our relationship is rare. I know sometimes
husbands can't handle it and they leave, but someone
told me that if the husband leaves, then chances are
he would have left anyway for something else. Before I

became chronically ill, and before it started appearing, I felt like I was more of the leader within the relationship. It's tricky having a husband who is also a caregiver. The two roles collide—for me at least. Not for him, but for me. It's not about the caregiver thing when it's just a normal marriage, and sometimes I have problems discerning between the two."

Nicole recognizes that her husband can sense what she needs and has taken on the leadership role to join her in caring for her health. "Actually, honestly, he knows what I need before I'll say it. Because he's here all the time, he can read me better than I can read myself sometimes, which aggravates me, haha!"

There are times when Nicole will want to push herself: "I'll want to do this, and do that, and do this, and do that, and go, and go, and go because in the moment I can do it. But it will hit me afterward with fatigue and irritability because I've overexerted myself. He'll see me and he'll urge me to slow down. I resent that, but in essence, it's helping me. At that moment, I don't know it; I can't see it. I can't appreciate it all."

It is difficult to go from strong independence and wanting to "go, and go, and go" to realizing that you need to slow down. Gratitude and frustration get wrapped together, which can be typical of any marriage. Reflecting on this, Nicole shares, "Sometimes I wonder if there should even be a separation. Am I aiming for something that shouldn't even be? Maybe it should just all fit together. I'm still working on that."

Relationships are work. Not just with spouses, but with friends and family too. I asked Nicole about how her relationships with others have changed. "Some family members have accepted it more than others. Some family members distance themselves because they don't know how to handle it, and I respect that." Nicole turned to a therapist to walk with her through this new territory. "My therapist told me that often family members, or people on the outside, have more problems adjusting to it than you do—than the person who has it. That saddens me because I feel like, 'I'm the one living through this. How dare you act like that toward me!' But my therapist helped me realize that sometimes it's harder for them to adjust than it is for the person who's living it, because the person who's living it doesn't have a choice; they have to live it."

As much as Nicole wants to be who she was before MS, her young nephew's acceptance helped her realize that she is so much more than her body. "He'll never know me walking, but I had to realize that doesn't matter to him. I'm Nicole . . . it doesn't matter that I can't walk or I can't run with him, or play with him, because all he wants to do is boy things anyway. It was a lesson I had to learn. At first it was so important [to me] for him to know I used to be able to do this, I used to be able to do that, but I had to evolve into realizing that it's all about who I am now, and who I am is going to shine through regardless, if I let it."

Recognizing that MS hasn't changed who she is at her core helped her to recognize all the capabilities she still has. "I can write. I can blog. I can advocate, and I can teach. I always feel like I'm wining this battle if I keep who I am. I'm a fun person. I'm a silly person. I like to laugh. I like to make people laugh, and if I can hold on to who I am, I feel like I am winning the battle regardless of if my legs listen to me or not. I'm winning the battle if I stay authentic to myself."

Nicole's most treasured support is in the simple efforts people make. "I like when people take the initiative to find out a little bit about MS and know that I'm not putting them off, I'm just really, really fatigued. I can't do all the activities that I used to do. I like when I'm physically respected." When Nicole began using a wheelchair, she discovered how far the support of respect goes. "I think riding in a wheelchair or scooter all the time plays on your self-esteem because people are always looking down on you. When people respect me, it makes a difference. It could be a stranger, or it could be a family member, or a friend who gives me human respect, human generosity."

Sometimes respect and generosity are lessons Nicole has realized she needs to help others learn. "A lot of times people in public don't know what to do. I think they need to be shown what to do. People have come up and patted me like I'm a child before. At first I was mad, but then I [thought] 'OK ,she just doesn't know, so it's my duty to educate her. She just doesn't know.'"

The biggest thing Nicole wants everyone to know is that she is still the same. "Just open the line of communication [with me], because once you hear me talk, once you see me, you'll say, 'Oh, OK, she's Nicole. She's just Nicole.' I went out to dinner with a friend of mine from college. I was nervous about seeing her because she hadn't seen me in a while. I knew she may have had an idea [of how I was doing], but she hadn't seen me. At the dinner, I said, 'Thank you for being so supportive and not freaking out or anything like that,' and she replied, 'Nicole, honestly, when I see you, you look the same, you weigh about the same, you're just Nicole!' I said 'Thank you!' All I could say was just 'Thank you!' I wished everybody knew that."

To help others recognize the ability and health she still has, Nicole is sure to present her image not as a sick person, but as someone vitally healthy. "Trying to be cute is important to me when I'm going places because I wear two big old braces on my legs when I'm in the wheelchair, so it affects my self-esteem. I try to look presentable as often as I can. I feel like if I look presentable it's an extra plus, and people know that everything is OK, that I'm all right, that I can still function."

Nicole's blog, "My New Normals" (*www.mynewnormals.com*) has proved to be an outlet to express her emotions and connect with others walking her same journey. Nicole had been blogging for a while before she realized that her parents were learning about how she was doing by reading her blog. She is now careful to give them a heads-up before she creates a new post. Even though it brings up some tough stuff, Nicole and her family see this outlet for self-expression as beneficial. "It's brought us closer because I think they understand it better. It's hard for me to talk to my mom about it because she has this way of looking at me. If she could take this from me and give it to herself, she would do it in a split second, and that is so heartfelt. I'm her daughter and I can respect that, so I try to call her beforehand and tell her things that I express on my blog. She said that she thinks the blog is good for me because that's the way I get my emotions out, and she's all for it."

For a woman with MS, neurologists (nervous system specialists) are a must. After testing out a few doctors, Nicole has found one who really supports her goals. "He's good. He's honest. He's not overly optimistic. I've had doctors say, 'Oh, this is gonna be it, this is gonna be the treatment. You're going to get better. You're going to be back running,' but that's not true. The doctor that I'm with now supports me, and he listens to me. [The doctors] know there's no cure. Whatever I want or whatever I ask for, they try their best to get it for me, and that makes me happy. I think in the end they want me to be happy because depression is secondary to MS." That type of support and honesty is crucial.

Nicole's smile tells you in a second that MS has done nothing to change the core of who she is. She works with her own expectations and strives to recognize her limitations to keep fatigue at bay. She continues to write and campaign for understanding and accessibility.

HEALTH TIPS

- It is important to have support as you process tough emotions and celebrate joys.

- Gather supporters who give you more energy than they take.

- Tackle financial stress by limiting expenses and utilizing resources available to bolster your income or assist with medical expenses.

- Include professionals that you trust on your support team.

- Ask for what you need with appreciation in a clear and direct way.

CHAPTER 7

Empower Yourself with Research

The temptation was overwhelming. I typed google.com into my Internet browser and stepped into a hypochondriac's dream. Once at Google's home page, the search bar begged for something interesting. My fingers clicked out "kidney disease and easily bruising." I'd had this bruise on my leg for a week. It wasn't dramatic, but I didn't remember how I had gotten it. I wanted Google to confirm my worst fears, that I was heading toward, or already in, kidney failure.

After my Portland doctor first mentioned the *T* word, I fueled my worries with a new pastime. I would watch for physical oddities and head to my diagnosing machine, a.k.a. the Internet, for a stranger to tell me that my health was careening down a steep decline. I was searching "kidney disease and shortness of breath," "kidney disease and fatigue," "kidney disease and symptoms," "kidney disease and transplant," and even "itching"— yes, "kidney disease and itching." Each search delivered hundreds of sites that predicted what my future would look like. I got to read stories about people whose kidneys were fine and then took a dramatic turn for the worse. I learned that I could develop a host of creepy symptoms as my body reacted to the toxins my kidney would eventually be unable to filter from my body.

Hours would go by as I got sucked into a world of pseudoscience that freaked me out. What started out as some mild fatigue and shortness of breath turned into exhaustion and a distinct tightness in my chest. I was playing mind games, and the Internet was winning. The more I searched, the worse I felt—and the more I wanted to search. I wasn't searching for how to become healthier, I was searching for how I was going to become sicker. And it was literally making me sick.

The New Pastime

The Internet has made it possible to effortlessly feed our worries. While some information is helpful, there are a ton of blogs, forums, articles, and news stories that can incite fear. When you start to feel off, it is way too easy to reach for the Internet to figure out what you've got and if dying is a possible side effect. This can easily lead to a cycle of symptom hawking.

Where I live, we constantly see hawks circling the sky looking for prey. With laser precision, they can see through tall grasses and dense forests for anything that moves. Like the hawk, we scan our bodies for anything out of the ordinary to feed the Internet. Especially with a new diagnosis, like I did with kidney disease, you can quickly do a number on your stress level by searching in this way.

When you start with one symptom, you usually come across a list of numerous other things to watch for and read about. Afternoons—heck, even days, can be spent doing one search after another. We have all become self-appointed medical experts.

There are lots of people out there who have opinions about every aspect of your treatment, and it is the vocal complainers who tend to post the most often. When things work, people don't feel the

> When you start to feel off, it is way too easy to reach for the Internet to figure out what you've got and if dying is a possible side effect. This can easily lead to a cycle of symptom hawking.

need to tell everyone; but if someone had a bad experience, they want to warn the world. That's why you get less of the feel-good stories and more of the freaky ones.

Only looking at the worst-case scenarios and searching every scratch, bump, or bruise you have is placing focus on things that are largely out of your control. You are an owner, and owners focus on what is in their control. Each search comes with a choice. You can choose to feed your worries or you can choose to feed your ability to heal.

Researching your health is about balance, obtaining knowledge without becoming obsessed. As soon as I began to search in healthy ways, I noticed that many of the symptoms I had been hawking went away.

Knowledge Gives Power

When you get diagnosed, you have to give much of your power away to doctors, medications, and unpredictable symptoms. Educating yourself about what is going on with your body and how to manage your health is a way to participate in your care. The unknown is scary because we assume that the slightest dusting of snow may cause an avalanche.

It is important to trust your health care team, but ultimately, you are responsible for your own care. You need all the power you can get, and knowledge delivers. Learning about your body enables you to:

- Provide clues toward your dse drug interactions.

- Seek a lifestyle that is beneficial for your health.

- Follow care plans.

- Explain what's going on to new members of your health care team.

- Understand when a symptom is of concern.

- Comprehend laboratory test results.

- Recognize health emergencies.

- Talk with your doctor about the benefits and risks of treatment.

- Mentally prepare for the future of coping with illness.

- Avoid harmful treatments.

- Prevent adverse drug interactions.

Before you understand your diagnosis, it can be easy to turn away from what is happening with your body. Ignoring the advice of your doctors and neglecting your health is counterproductive. Denial breeds all sorts of excuses as to why you don't need to change your diet, start exercising, or take the medication prescribed. This type of fear masquerades as hope that if you pretend things are as they used to be, maybe they will be. Learning the facts of your illness can be scary, but it also helps you woman-up and take care of what needs to be taken care of. That is power.

> Learning the facts of your illness can be scary, but it also helps you woman-up and take care of what needs to be taken care of. That is power.

Know Your Medical History

I am continually surprised when a doctor commends me on how much I know about my medical history. What's the big deal? Doesn't everyone know this? I shouldn't be the anomaly. It should be normal for every woman to know the details of her health. Finding a diagnosis and treating an illness is like putting a puzzle together, a puzzle that you provide most of the pieces for. If you have lost a few pieces, the picture the doctor is looking for will not come into view. A missing puzzle piece could lead to receiving inappropriate, and potentially dangerous, treatment. Physicians tag team a lot, especially if you are cared for at a teaching hospital where residents and interns come and go. The days of the family doctor who treats everyone in town and has known you since you were born are rare. Computer systems have made medical records more accessible, but in my experience nothing beats personally knowing what a new doctor needs to be aware of.

Understanding my medical history and current health status has proved vital on several occasions. One year around Christmas my grandmother had a fall and was in critical condition in the ICU. Phillip and I flew down to be with my mom. Leading up to our last-minute visit, I had been coughing and had a few episodes of being out of breath. It felt like my lungs were glued together, and forcing air in was tough. One afternoon, we had lunch with some good friends who lived in the area, and Phillip and I both noticed that I was getting out of breath just holding a conversation. I was concerned, but I wasn't running a fever and didn't feel sick. I am also stubborn; I was there to support my grandmother, not to see a doctor myself. The evening after our lunch, Phillip and I were on our way back from visiting my grandmother when he decided he'd had enough of hearing me cough, and we were going to urgent care to see what was going on with my lungs.

After the nurse practitioner listened to my lungs she assessed that I probably had bronchitis, and she needed to prescribe antibiotics to fight the infection. Kidneys process everything that ends up in our blood, including medications. This meant that I would need an adjusted dose of the drug so as to not overwhelm my kidney. Because I knew the exact value of my latest lab results, I was able to give that to the nurse practitioner and the on-call kidney specialist to get my prescription dosage correct. That was not the first time I'd had to assist an urgent care doctor with prescribing the correct dose of a new medication. The bronchitis I had that Christmas turned out to be the pneumonia and the collapsed lung mentioned in chapter 5. When Phillip and I found ourselves in the ER after returning home from visiting my grandmother, knowing my health status helped hospital staff quickly provide tests and treatments while protecting my kidney function.

Doctors and nurses have a lot on their plate. Many work long shifts that add up to between sixty and eighty hours per week.[25] That is a lot of patients to see. Your doctor has an amazing memory to have passed all of his school exams, but charts can become quite thick, and expecting that the doctor will have reviewed everything before he sees you is unrealistic. You won't need to give a twenty-minute dissertation on every ache, sneeze, and hangnail you've ever had, but knowing the basics is important. Be prepared to share with your doctor:

- Your available family health history, including major diseases such as heart disease, diabetes, lung disease, Alzheimer's, rheumatoid arthritis, hypertension, and cancer

- Your past and current medications with dosages, frequency, and when you took what last

- Past and current diagnosis

- How your symptoms have changed over time

- Adverse drug reactions, including allergies to any medications

- Past surgeries

- Past hospitalizations

- Possible causes of your diagnosis

---

25 E. Ray Dorsey, MD, MBA, David Jarjoura, PhD, and Gregory W. Rutecki, MD. "Influence of Controllable Lifestyle on Recent Trends in Specialty Choice by US Medical Students," *JAMA 2003*; 290 (9):1173–78.

- Current treatment plan

- Physical abnormalities

- Known genetic abnormalities

- Lifestyle changes over time, including diet, exercise, smoking, and drug and alcohol use

- Mental health diagnosis and history

- Immunizations

- Major accidents

Become a researcher of your own quirks. Check in with your body to begin learning what is normal for you and what is out of the ordinary. Doctors cannot read your mind. You need to speak up when something is important for your care. And please don't be embarrassed. They've seen it all; goodness knows I've horrified a few medical staff in my day. The better you know your body, the better the doctor will be able to help.

Internet Advice

You can have your first blog post up in less than an hour. Anyone can immediately become an expert on the Internet, and many do. For diseases A through Z, there is a host of people who are happy to give you their advice about your treatment—some for free, some for a "Very Low One-Time Fee of $59.99!"

It can be beneficial to be connected to a group of people who are coping with your same illness, but treating their recommendations as you would an MD's is risky. People on the Internet are strangers. They have not examined you and do not know your unique symptoms.

Look at the people you meet on the Internet as friends, not experts. Your friends give you advice, they listen, they understand, they get it, but you also know that they are your peers and do not have the training of your medical team.

My shortness of breath while attempting to trek the Austrian mountains was not unusual for me. When I was in school, I always wondered why I finished running the mile last. I didn't have anything that appeared to be hindering my level of physical fitness, but shortly after take-off I'd be gasping and need to walk to the finish. People had mentioned over the years that it sounds like I wheeze when I talk, but I'd never paid much attention.

During a routine checkup my doctor thought that I had asthma because he too heard the wheezing. We tried inhalers and antihistamines, but I was still getting out of breath on exertion. Tests were ordered that indicated I had decreased lung capacity, but the cause remained a mystery. I was poked and prodded, and we still had no answers.

I decided to jump on the VACTERL forum online and ask if anyone had experienced shortness of breath as part of VACTERL. There it was, something I had not thought of. A few people commented that they observed similar symptoms caused by scoliosis, and my version of VACTERL does include scoliosis.

> By all means, receive input; but bring what you are reading to the attention of your medical team so they can help you sort through the good-for-you stuff and the just-trying-to-freak-you-out stuff.

On my next visit to the lung specialist I mentioned scoliosis. The doctor concurred that it could impact my breathing. I began to see a chiropractor and do yoga, which somewhat helped to open my lungs.

By all means, receive input; but bring what you are reading to the attention of your medical team so they can help you sort through the good-for-you stuff and the just-trying-to-freak-you-out stuff. Experimenting with your own health is OK if your medical team is aware of your experiments. Your doctor coordinates your care, and that can be hard if you are secretly trying the Internet's Magic Cure for What Ails You while also trying your doctor's recommendations. Be consistent and transparent.

Doing the Research

There are a number of credible online sources that you can consider the University of Your Health. Supplement conversations with your doctor and learn more about your body by rolling up your sleeves and digging into the good, and technical, stuff. Researching from this perspective is less sensationalized. Rather than feeding worry, you are feeding yourself knowledge of the latest research by some of the brightest minds in medicine.

Be sure the source of your research speaks to its credibility. Here's what to look for:

- The author's professional credentials. The most common credentials for mainstream health practitioners are: MD, PhD, MS, PA, and RN. All indicate a level of professional training that has been verified by an accredited educational institution.

- Studies conducted through health research institutes at universities or university hospitals.

- Articles or books obtained through a medical library.

- Studies published in professional journals. Two of the most famous are *The Journal of the American Medical Association* (JAMA) and *The New England Journal of Medicine* (NEJM). Researchers must have their work reviewed by peers in their specialty to have it accepted for publication. Jumping through these hoops ensures quality and accuracy.

- Studies that are cited by other studies. Professional articles end with citations of books and articles that have informed the current research. Articles that are frequently cited are held in higher regard within the research community.

- Studies promoted by professional associations such as the American Heart Association, the American Cancer Society, the National Kidney Foundation, or the American Diabetes Association. For a complete list of associations visit: *www.healthfinder.gov.* Click the link on the left, "Find Services and Information." Toward the bottom of the page, you will see a link for "Find a Health Organization."

One phenomenal source for medical research is the United States National Library of Medicine, the world's largest medical library, which can be accessed online at: *www.pubmed.gov.* There is a quick start guide on the home page which will walk you through how to search for your specific condition or symptom. It is easy to use and will deliver lists of pertinent articles for you to spend an afternoon with. Each article has an abstract, a summary of the research conducted, and the conclusions reached. If a certain article's abstract piques your interest, you can search for the full text. PubMed does not house the full text, but where available they link to the article's full text at the publisher's website. Many articles are free.

Remember libraries? Has it been a while since you visited your local library? They are still there and are eager to help you find what you're looking for. Many libraries stock professional journals, and some even participate in interlibrary loan programs where they can obtain books from larger library systems outside your own. And it's all free! Who doesn't love that?

If scholarly research isn't your thing, there are other ways to learn about your diagnosis. WebMD (*www.webmd .com*) is a good source for easy-to-understand medical information. You can research symptoms or diseases and receive information about possible diagnoses, treatments, and side effects. Their site has a medical review board which helps inspect the accuracy of the information and keeps a pulse on current health research. You can also visit the Mayo Clinic website (*www.mayoclinic.com*). They are one of the best health care facilities in the United States and maintain a website that allows you to search for all sorts of health information. It too has a symptom checker and information on countless diseases and conditions.

Going directly to one of these sites ensures that the information you are getting is reliable. Search engines, such as Google, Yahoo, and Bing, use formulas that do not take into account the qualifications of a website's author. The top listings for any given search are based on relevancy and popularity, not necessarily scientific scrutiny.

You can also ask your doctor to recommend supplemental reading, and she will point you in the right direction.

Now what to avoid. I choose to stay away from sales letters. There is a new Internet trend that has proved effective where single page websites are created with the sole purpose of selling something. I'm sure you've seen these impossibly long sites with numerous testimonials and promise after promise of the miracle cure that can be at your fingertips if you just get out your credit card. They are intriguing. They are hopeful. You know you want to be one of those smiling people who used to suffer terribly from a disease until you discovered this approach and now not only is the disease cured, but so are your relationship and financial problems. I always wonder, if this really is a miracle cure why hasn't my doctor heard about it yet? Perplexing.

If you find that you are getting lost in the details or that you have tipped the scales toward the obsessed, take a

> If you find that you are getting lost in the details or that you have tipped the scales toward the obsessed, take a break. Grab a cup of tea. Pet the dog. Take a walk. Relax.

break. Grab a cup of tea. Pet the dog. Take a walk. Relax. Then gather together things that seem promising or interesting and compile a list of questions for your doctor.

Become a Research Subject

I had never met a doctor who knew so much about VACTERL Association. Typically, I hear, "Yeah, I think I remember reading about that in a medical textbook." I was at the National Institutes of Health (NIH), where Dr. Benjamin Solomon was researching the possible causes of VACTERL Association. His interest in VACTERL started during his pediatric rotation where he happened to see an abnormally high number of VACTERL cases. He sensed the families' frustration of wanting to understand why their child was born needing extensive surgeries and facing lifelong challenges, and he wanted to find answers.

When I was born, VACTERL was so new it was only called VATER Association. The additional letters were added later as doctors began to recognize consistent cardiac involvement. Back in 1979, my diagnosis was pieced together with X-rays as one thing was discovered after another. My family was learning together with my doctors.

When I heard about Dr. Solomon's research, I jumped at the chance to participate. Meeting a doctor who knew more about VACTERL than I did was a gift. I was fascinated to learn things that I didn't know about my body. Phillip and I spent a week in Washington, DC visiting the hospital in the morning to have ultrasounds, X-rays, lab work, EKGs, genetic counseling, and physical exams. Dr. Solomon and his team were putting together a picture of my unique manifestation of VACTERL. Once they confirmed that I was indeed "classic" VACTERL, my DNA was extracted to be analyzed against other patients in the study.

While I had been confident that scoliosis was the culprit of my shortness of breath, I learned that in fact many children born with an abnormal connection between their trachea and esophagus (tracheoesophageal fistula [TEF], the *T* and *E* in VACTERL) have asthma-like symptoms in their larger bronchial tubes that doesn't respond to traditional asthma treatments. This small piece of knowledge took a huge weight off my back. I had always felt lazy, and subsequently guilty, for not having the physical endurance of my peers. Knowing that the best course of action for my lungs was to recognize my limits allowed for the self-compassion I had long been denied.

I also learned that in addition to scoliosis, I had some vertebral abnormalities that explained my back pain and difficulty maintaining proper posture—another source of personal guilt. Participating in the research helped me to understand by body better, and I came away from NIH a more sensitive steward of my health.

There are numerous types of research to participate in. There are studies similar to mine, where they profile diseases and conditions to search for a cause. There are studies that test new medications and treatments, studies that look at how various behaviors impact health, and studies that investigate the mind-body connection.

There will be lots of things to mull over, depending on the type of study you're considering. Since the research that I participated in involved DNA, I had to decide if I wanted to know if I was genetically predisposed to certain conditions, such as cancer or Alzheimer's. Studies that test new drugs have a variety of risks since the side effects and outcome may be uncertain for humans, depending on where the drug is at in the testing process. If you look into becoming a research subject, be sure to have a thorough conversation with the research team to understand the risks and benefits of participation.

To find studies that are recruiting research participants, go to: *www.clinicaltrials.gov.* You will find a link on the home page to search for clinical trials based on research topic and location. The search feature will return a list of trials and indicate if they are recruiting, completed, terminated, or not yet recruiting. Click on the link to a trial you are interested in, and the purpose of the study, location, researchers, participant profile, contacts, and other pertinent information, including related scholarly articles, will come up. What's better than reading the research? Being the research.

Research Wellness

In addition to researching the technical stuff, spend some time researching your wellness. Look into diet, exercise, meditation, mindfulness techniques, yoga, qigong, and other interesting modalities. Illness is a prompting not just to cure what's wrong, but to elevate your total health.

As a general rule, I give new practices a one- to three-month trial period. After that, I evaluate if my new habit is working and keep going or drop it. Remember to look at these practices with the same scrutiny as you do your medical care. For instance, if the doctor on the cover of the diet book looks like he could use a diet, move on. I also get turned off if the answer to a guru's "secret formula" for wellness comes only after three easy installments of $199 each.

There are literally thousands of practices you could try. Don't do too many at once or you'll get interference and won't know if going sugar-free or yoga has decreased your inflammation. Your intuition will guide you to what is next on your wellness journey; honor her wisdom.

Absolute versus "Statistically Significant"

In research, there is a difference between a "statistically significant" result and an absolute. In statistics, "statistically significant" means that something is most likely not due to chance. If you read a study where a "statistically significant" number of people had a bad reaction to a treatment, this does not mean that you absolutely will. Similarly, just because Suzie on the forum is complaining about a massive headache she got after starting a new medication does not mean that your body will react the same way to the same medication. The reverse is also true. Someone could have a reversal of their symptoms by only drinking ginger tea, but that does not mean that it will work for everyone.

It can be hard to get your hopes up about new things you are discovering only to find that your body doesn't respond the way you wish it would. Six months before I started the transplant testing, I went super strict with my diet. I wasn't sure if it would reverse things, but based on some books I'd read, I had hope. When I found out that my kidney function had declined, I pouted all the way to the cupcake shop. The next day I went back to a healthy diet, but this time with a bit more leeway for impromptu pizza night.

Health is trial and error. Unless something is absolute, and very little is, the attitude to have is openness. Try new things, get creative, explore and learn, but remain open about what the results may be in your oh-so-unique body.

Your Health Binder

As you gather research and doctor visits become as frequent as visits to your hairdresser, you'll want to keep all of your information in a safe place. This place is your health binder, and it is essential. It is easy to keep organized and easy to transport.

Time for a fun-run to your local office supply store. You'll need:

- A binder

- A glitzy pen

- Hole-punched ruled paper

- Hole-punched folders

- A hole-punched business card holder

- Dividers

You can cover the front of your binder with a collage of inspiring images or quotes to disguise all the sterile medical stuff you're about to collect.

Here's what goes inside:

- Your medical history—a bullet-pointed narrative of your major stuff and your family's major stuff.

- Contact information of medical professionals—this is what the business card holder is for.

- Lab and other test results—I never leave an appointment without a copy of my results for my binder.

- Research—articles, blog posts, book recommendations, clinical trial summaries, and anything you'd want to ask about or show your doctor.

- List of your current and past medications with side effect sheets—new medications come from the pharmacy with a list of side effects and other information. Hole-punch these and keep them in your binder. When that weird rash shows up, you'll want to know if it was caused by the pill you just swallowed.

- Health journal—use the hole-punched ruled paper to create a health journal. You can track your diet, exercise, symptoms, drug reactions, blood pressure, and mental health.

- Notes—keep some blank pages in your notebook to jot down notes at the doctor's office about new care plans or things to watch for.

- List of questions—before each doctor visit, compile a list of questions and concerns so that you don't get back home and think "ugh, I meant to ask about that burning sensation."

Because Phillip and I have moved every few years, my health binder has been invaluable to inform new doctors of my health history and status. Before I meet a new physician, I make a copy of my past medical records (all the way back to when I was born) and come in with some "light" reading for them to do.

Your medical records are yours; just because they are housed in a doctor's office does not mean that you are not entitled to copies. Many offices are happy to provide this for you, but my mom and I did have to stage a sit-in once to get some records that a receptionist did not feel like copying. I have referenced those records many times and am glad we waited.

A Conversation with Sharmyn McGraw, Researcher Extraordinaire and Cushing's Disease Speaker

Sharmyn McGraw researched her way to a diagnosis of Cushing's disease. She is a professional speaker and supporter of patients coping with hormone disorders and has been featured on *Mystery Diagnosis* and *The Montel Williams Show*. Visit her at: *www.hormones411.org*.

"I stopped sleeping at night, anxiety started building, I had a round moon face, my hair—long, thick, blonde hair—fell out in handfuls, and I had a rash starting to cover my body. My stomach stuck out like I was pregnant with twins. One time, when I was waiting to see my doctor, one of the mothers in the office said, 'Oh, when's your baby due?' I was so humiliated. I had to say, 'Oh, I'm not pregnant, I'm just overweight.' I remember thinking how sad inside that made me because I had been a size 2. This went on for seven years, me just searching for answers to my health issues. The more health issues I got, the more doctors would blame me, and the more society blamed me. 'What is she doing? Why is she doing this to herself?' Inside I was looking at the world just drifting by me and constantly thinking, 'When is someone going to recognize what is medically wrong with me?'"

Over a period of one year, Sharmyn gained one hundred pounds at the same time she was working out five nights per week. At age thirty-one, doctors initially thought she had symptoms of premenopause and treated her with antidepressants. Despite the medication, her anxiety increased and her symptoms grew worse. Sharmyn reached her breaking point.

"Eventually I realized that I didn't believe the medical community was going to help me. I knew I wasn't going to live much longer. I could barely walk anymore.

I couldn't even remember a simple sentence. My facial structure had changed so much that I didn't even recognize myself in the mirror. I literally could not see who I was in there; that person in the mirror was not me, it was not the person I knew. I couldn't walk up stairs anymore without holding on to a rail and taking one stair at a time. I couldn't sleep more than fifteen minutes at night. I honestly knew I was not going to live another year. At that point something kicked in, and I thought, "Go pull every medical record that you can."

Sharmyn began collecting her records from the many, many doctors she had seen over the last seven years. She recalls, "I just sat for hours. I read doctors' notes and things like that. Something in my heart kept saying, 'This is a hormone; keep searching.' And then I found this word, *cortisol.*"

She took to the Internet and had a life-changing moment. "One night I realized, 'Oh my gosh, they've missed it. I have a pituitary brain tumor!' It was this research that saved her life.

After seven years of searching, at first Sharmyn questioned if she really had found her own answer. "How could it be this simple? All these medical doctors, naturopaths, everybody I had sought help from, psychiatrists and therapists, everybody had blamed me, but no one knew about this disease? It was called Cushing's disease."

She knew she had an answer, and she was determined to have her researched confirmed. She sought out the best experts she could find on Cushing's disease and began to learn even more. Sharmyn found out that Cushing's disease is a secondary disease to a pituitary brain tumor. She dug in deeper to figure out why it took so long for her to be diagnosed with a disease that had such a broad impact on her life. "Cushing's disease is specific to a tumor in the pituitary gland, and the pituitary gland controls your whole quality of life. It's our master plan. It regulates all of our hormones. The problem is, we don't have much research on it, and most doctors were historically trained very little about it because they believed that it is a rare disorder."

Since her diagnosis and successful surgery to remove the tumor eleven years ago, Sharmyn, along with neurosurgeon and Cushing's expert Dr. Daniel Kelly, have been on a mission to educate the public and the medical community to help others avoid the anguish she went through.

After Sharmyn's story began airing on *Mystery Diagnosis* she discovered just how many people could relate to what she has gone through. "Still to this day, I get e-mail, after e-mail, after e-mail of people thanking me that I gave them their life back. Because of that one show, they got a correct diagnosis, and otherwise they would've probably died."

> This disease forced me to see what was real about me and what I had dreamed up about me. I found that I was a much stronger person than I had ever given myself credit for.

One blessing that came out of Sharmyn's journey was confidence. "I went through this disease not knowing what was wrong with me. It really changed me inside. It forced me to see what was real about me and what I had dreamed up about me. I found that I was a much stronger person than I had ever given myself credit for."

Her newfound self-esteem and passion to help others pushed Sharmyn past prior struggles with dyslexia to begin writing. "Even though I'm dyslexic, I can still be taught. I still have the thoughts and the passion to help people. I thought, 'If I'm going to help people on a bigger scale, I'm going to have to get over the fear of writing.' I took a class on how to write for magazines." With the help of her writing teacher, Sharmyn began submitting query letters to magazines about sharing her story. "I sent it out to over thirteen magazines, and I got rejections: 'Thank you very much, but no thank you.' I never gave up because the passion was so strong; nothing else mattered to me."

Ultimately, Sharmyn was invited to write her story and have it published in *Woman's Day* magazine. From there, things took off, and she was able to begin helping other patients on a much larger scale. "I didn't know which was more exciting, and more fulfilling—to know that my article would go out to millions of people who would find out about Cushing's, or that I was actually a writer. I've really learned that it only takes one person to believe in themselves; then others will believe in you."

Sharmyn's passion and research continued to grow over the years. Out of her experience, she has become a respected and assertive patient. "I tell other patients, if you're with a doctor who doesn't give you respect, get another one, because these guys are the top of the world. They treat their patients with respect. They learn from their patients. They're there to care about their patients and to help improve medicine. If you have a physician who doesn't take a team approach and hear you out, get another one. I lay it on the line when I first go in: This is who I am. This is what I expect, and this is what I'm willing to do. I'm willing to do what you say as long as I understand why you're saying it, and as long as you understand where I'm coming from in my life."

When she finds a doctor who doesn't seem to care or treat her with respect, rather than just silently walk away, she takes a direct approach with an aim of improving the doctor's practice. "Even though some people think

I'm crazy, so what. I actually write the doctor a letter and explain to him why our working relationship didn't work. I say it very professionally. I make sure that I'm not accusatory. I just go about it like a colleague would explain it to them. I've had some doctors tell me thank you, because they need to help other patients, and they'll go about it a different way next time. I take care to empower and validate myself. I deserve good health care, and I deserve a working relationship with my medical professional, just like I would if I hired a vendor to do work at my house."

After cycling through doctor after doctor to figure out why she was gaining weight and becoming more ill, Sharmyn has gained the courage to get to know the credentials of the medical professionals she works with. "We go to doctors all the time and think, 'Great, they went to medical school.' We don't know what medical school, we don't know how well they did in medical school, and, to be quite frank, we're not even really allowed to ask. You kind of understand that if they earned it, they're probably very good. They may understand their profession, but we don't. We don't even so much as look on the wall to see what their degrees are in. We put so much trust in a doctor that an insurance company approved. I want a doctor who is going to be honest with me, work with me, and get me healthy, so I don't have to keep going to doctors."

With all of her experience researching Cushing's and other hormonal disorders, I asked Sharmyn, "What are your best tips for researching personal health?" She started with the first place we all go: the Internet. "I think the Internet is good. It's an excellent source, but I would be very careful about what you're reading. If you don't understand what you're reading, bring it with you to the doctor and have them explain.

Another thing is, be open to other ideas, too. I like to combine Eastern and Western medicine. I just recently started doing yoga again. It has strengthened my core so much, and I started feeling good again. Surround yourself with things other than just medical journals. Research on yoga and Pilates has been beneficial, and if you can't do those things, research what you can do. Research how much laughter helps people. Rent funny movies; that could be research. Research what ten funny movies you're going to watch for the next two weeks. Also find out what they're doing in other countries. Find out what they're doing in other hospitals. Find out what they are doing on the East Coast. Find out what they are doing on the West Coast. And don't take everything [as] 'this is exactly what's going to happen.' Not everything is an exact science. Be open to newer ideas, or different ideas. Really be open-minded to more than one idea about how to get better."

Going from a size 2 to 250 pounds and researching her way back to health taught Sharmyn about the deeper side of people. "It changed my whole life; it changed my acceptance of who I am. Now I look at people with such com-passion. I don't judge people by their cover. You don't know what someone's story is. That's the biggest thing that I'm proud of, that it changed the inside of me. I like who I am inside."

> I don't judge people by their cover. You don't know what someone's story is.

Sharmyn lives in Southern California, where she facilitates the pituitary patient support group through Saint John's Brain Tumor Center at the John Wayne Cancer Institute. She continues to speak, write, and spread her message of becoming an advocate for oneself.

HEALTH TIPS

- Find balance between learning about your health and becoming a hot, worried mess.

- Check the credibility of the information you find online.

- Consider participating in a research study by visiting *clinicaltrials.gov.*

- Keep an open mind that you may not react to a certain medication or treatment in the same way others do.

- Maintain a health binder to keep everything organized.

CHAPTER 8

Live What Needs to Be Lived Today

On occasion, I have been known to stomp around the house gathering Icy Hot and heating pads when my back has decided it has had enough of standing upright. Pain is no fun. It grips you at your core and prevents any rational decision-making. The thing is, I know when the pain is coming, and much to my chagrin my mind becomes obsessed with preventing it, which always guarantees that I will reach the tipping point of having a full blown *episode*.

I have had this back pain every few months since I was thirteen, a well-ingrained pattern. It was once caused by a wayward drop of rain that slipped down the back of my shirt. At that first slight pinch or bit of soreness, I become fixated on trying to prevent what I assume is coming. I know, as Phillip reminds me, that in my desperation to avoid pain I am just making it worse.

Phillip and I always take a trip for our anniversary. We got the idea from close friends of ours, and it is a cherished tradition. We usually get away somewhere close for a night or two, but for our fifth anniversary we had two free flights and decided to go to New York and drive up through Vermont to see the fall foliage.

I felt great while we were in the city doing the touristy stuff. I felt great when we rented the car. Felt great in the Catskill Mountains, great at the Baseball Hall of Fame. Great when we arrived at the Vermont bed and breakfast. And then . . . I felt "the twinge," a millisecond pinch in the left side of my back just below my shoulder blade. I tried to ignore it, but already my mind was in emergency mode: Oh my goodness, what if my back is going to go out? Not now, *please* not now.

I futilely tried to relax and felt the pinch again. I believed I could prevent the third pinch if I twisted my left arm around to massage the muscle that had started to spasm. I know that rubbing my back just makes me anxious and worry more, but I do it anyway. Over breakfast, Phillip sees me eating with one hand and has caught on to my preoccupation. I am terrified that things will get worse to the point that spasms come every few seconds, making every twist, step, and bump of the car ride a prompt for stabbing pain. I am already remembering the times before, how the one-millisecond twinge can turn into massive spasms on both sides of my spine. I am even more scared that I forgot to pack pain medication. This is not how this trip is supposed to go!

What were just two twinges became massive muscle spasms in my mind before my body ever went there. The stress felt over "what could happen" makes it happen. Thirty minutes after the first twinge, things are going downhill and we are headed to the store for Icy Hot, a heating pad, and an adapter that will allow me to plug everything into the car. I slept and missed the foliage from Vermont through Massachusetts. I woke up in our next hotel room with Phillip at the edge of the bed, take-out dinner in hand. It was a bad day.

Where Do Your Thoughts Live Most of the Time?

Illness comes with a thousand small triggers like this. There is the new rash that just showed up, the odd pain in your hip, the list of fifty side effects that your new medication is known to cause, the shortness of breath you have when you walk up the stairs, and the story you just saw on the news about someone who is battling an illness with symptoms that now seem eerily similar to yours. The mind loves this type of juicy fodder. It can spend hours weaving dreadful scenarios that never seem to feature you as the heroine. It does this because that is our mind's job. The problem is that even though your new medication is not likely to give you both diarrhea and constipation, plus depression, hemorrhaging, and blurred vision, your mind assumes it might.

Aside from the grandiose hats, there is a lot to analyze in horse racing. A horse's age, its past performance, who its trainer is, who the jockey is, the length of the race, your risk tolerance, and, of course, that its name is "I'll Have Another." Even with all that, you still don't know which horses will come in first, second, and third. It is all speculation, a game. When you get sick, like a gambler playing the ponies, the mind races around scrutinizing all of your available information: What does this remind you of? What does the Internet tell you about your symptoms? Who have you known who has had this? What does your doctor say? It uses this information to make an estimate about the future. That prediction tells you how stressed you should be right now. The mind is a computer calculating the odds to tell you how to place your bet. But this, too, is just speculation.

When the horses leave the gate each hoof on the ground is the only thing that matters until they cross the finish line. With you, how your health is at this moment is the only thing that's real. The mind is designed to jump from the past to the future. Its job is to think up stories of how things were and how things might be. It's all these what-ifs that make us stressed.

As the horses race to the finish, it's rare for your mind to be in lockstep with them. Even in the moment, your mind is thinking, "Ugh, I should have bet on number twenty-seven." Then it jumps to, "If my horse can stay in the lead, I'll make $150." And it continues to bounce another fifteen places before the race is over. With all the bouncing around, you miss the elegance of the race.

It is super easy to get caught up in our thoughts and overanalyze things such as: What happens if this drug doesn't work? What if my digestive system can't handle the Mexican restaurant my co-workers just pulled up at? Yet, if we can separate ourselves from the chatter, we can better manage our present reality rather than live a life made anxious by the mind's incessant speculation.

Being Present

On a recent hike through the mountains, my dad and I met a mountain biker who was on an insane ride down the bouldered trail we were hiking up. His ride was an intense exercise in remaining present. He had laser focus to maneuver his bike between and over sharp rocks that threatened his balance at every turn. If he started day-dreaming about what he was going to have for dinner, he would have surely missed a rock and been headed for the ER. He knew he was being crazy. He was also one of the most alive people I've ever met. Though we talked for less than a minute, I could see it in his eyes.

This is why people do extreme sports. It forces them into the present moment, out of their heads and into their body, into the action of life. They have no time to analyze their experience because they have to be actively in their experience.

When your mind wanders off into a stressful place, you can guide it back to the present, without careening down a mountain on a bike. We can't unlearn how to contemplate the future, nor would we want to, but we can practice bringing ourselves back into the present with two questions:

- What are the facts of my situation? (The who, what, when, where, and how.)

- How do I feel about those facts? (The joy, pain, gratitude, fear, happiness, and frustration.)

Grab your journal and answer these two questions for how you are doing right now. I'll wait.

ASK YOURSELF

- What are the facts of my situation?

- How do I feel about those facts?

Make note of any items that relate to the past or future.

All finished? Read back over your answers and notice if you inserted any thoughts about the past or the future. For instance, right now I am:

- Sitting on my deck. My dog, Abbey, is panting. My butt is numb from the weight of the laptop and the way I'm slouching in the chair. I can feel the sun on my feet. I have to pee. A blackbird is chattering.

- I feel a bit anxious, but when I look up and see the trees I feel content. I have health issues but am not currently in pain.

If I had added in "my back might go out" or "I bet my kidney will be worse at my upcoming appointment," I would have been bringing the future into my moment on the deck. While that future is probable, it is not true at this moment, and thinking about it would take away from being outside with Abbey. Don't let your illness steal your moments; it has already taken e.n.o.u.g.h.

It is rare that we notice the details of our surroundings and emotions without trying to analyze our way out of experiencing them. "What are the facts?" and "How do I feel?" are the two key questions to make sure you are aware of what is in front of you.

I have had lots of practice trying to stay present through pain since my fated Icy Hot drive through New England. Phillip and I were recently back in Lake Tahoe with some relatives for a getaway. I spent one day walking all over town looking in shop windows and taking in the scenery. That evening, I could tell that I overdid it. We went to see a comedian, and while everyone laughed, I cringed and silently begged my back to not go out. I started my well-worn routine of worry and furiously rubbing at the impending pain. By the time we left the next morning, history had repeated itself and I was in full-spasm mode. Through breakfast and goodbyes, I winced at the little man with the very sharp knife stabbing me in the back.

By the time Phillip and I got in the car, it would be another two hours before I would be at home with pain relievers. Yes, I forgot them . . . again. As the engine started I closed my eyes, leaned back hard into my seat, and focused with everything I had on the moments between the pain. "Right now I feel OK . . . still OK . . . breathe . . . doing good . . . breathe . . . still good. Relax . . . breathe . . ." I kept coming back to the present. I refused to let my mind jump forward to the next impending pain. I refused to think about the bumps and curves in the road that could exacerbate things. I just focused on how my muscles felt in each moment, and my back was calm for the two-hour ride home. After it had spasmed every few seconds for the last twelve hours, it was completely calm, without Icy Hot, without heating pads set to high, without painkillers. It was calm.

You can come to the present at any point when you are getting fearful about your future. This is especially helpful before big medical tests, such as MRIs or lab work. Just ask, "What are the facts? How do I feel?" You might find that your answer is something along the lines of "I am having a biopsy accompanied by lots of fearful thoughts about the future." That too is a fact. Noticing what your mind is doing—having fearful thoughts—without leaping into the future with them is empowering. You can watch your mind work without getting caught up in the tension those thoughts produce.

A Good Day

Synonymous with illness are good days and bad days. Actually, synonymous with life are good days and bad days.

The few years we lived in Portland, Phillip and I were close to the small coastal kite-wielding town Phillip grew up in. The Pacific Northwest, and specifically the weather, was familiar to my husband. In preparation for our move there, he told me that it was going to be cold, rainy, and gray *all* of the time. I was ready to hunker down and never see the sun again. There are a lot of rainy days in Oregon, but the sun does shine there too. Beautiful, glistening sun. Since a lot of time is spent indoors, while the sun is out, you better get your butt outside to enjoy it. I found that I took more walks and sat outside more in Oregon than I ever did in California. Rather than despise the rain, I was grateful for it because it created a gorgeous landscape of forests and creeks. The rain made the sun that much more enjoyable.

How often do we let the good days pass us by because we are too busy to notice them? When we feel good, we rush from here to there doing laundry and running errands before a bad day sneaks up on us. We only see the bad days as permission to pay attention to our personal needs. Good days tend to be for everyone else.

Back in chapter 3, we talked about life as a wheel, and the wheel is not just your illness. It is also comprised of your career, friends and family, romance, personal growth, recreation, environment, and finances. Yes, on bad days, your focus is mainly health. But good days are the days for the rest of your life. Good days are the Oregon sun. Use the time to focus on your projects and the things you enjoy to balance out the drudgery of pain and fatigue.

Good days are the Mardi Gras of being sick. Yes, you may have to fit in picking up the dry cleaning, but also take time to paint, swing in the park, or bake your favorite cake. Bad days seem a bit less bad when you are maximizing your good days not just for chores, but for the stuff that causes you to laugh uncontrollably and hug everyone around you.

A Bad Day

Oh, dear, sweet Dr. Hendren. I mentioned his surprising call to check in on me in the last chapter. I was nine years old at my last appointment with Dr. Hendren. He was in California for something or another, and my mom took me for a visit. He wanted to inspect my muscle tone and how his work had healed over the years, but in order to do so I would need to be under general anesthesia . . . the day after my ninth birthday. When you are little, birthdays are sacred. I was irrationally pissed, and in my anger I swatted at my doctor. I'm sure my mom told me to get a grip, but I know my bottom lip was out a mile and my face was wet with tears.

I'm not suggesting you hit your doctor. I was a brat, and what I did was embarrassingly wrong. However, there is a lesson in there. The day I got the news that I'd have to go under was a bad day, and my little nine-year-old self let it be a bad day. If you don't feel well, be present with that. If you're in the fetal position crying on the floor, be present with that. If you're angry, go into an open field and yell and be present with your anger. The tension to push back from how we're feeling, physically and emotionally, is stressful.

What if you gave yourself permission to have a bad day? What would it be like to check in with yourself in the morning and actually listen to what your body is telling you? What if you were present with your bad day? What would it be like to embrace it with open arms, to understand that your body needs a rest, and to honor that without judgment?

What if you gave yourself permission to have a bad day?

Meeting the moment in this way helps you release stress. Rather than exacerbate stress by thinking up more things to worry about, you sink into what's really going on, what you're feeling. Give yourself permission to feel what fear or sadness or pain feels like.

I think that the positive thinking movement is wonderful in a lot of ways, but it has also divorced us from our painful emotions, and those suckers don't go away on their own without feeling them first. You are allowed to have days that are not all sunshine and flowers. It does rain too.

What's fascinating about the rain is that when you stand out in it, you see it for what it is. You can accept it. The whole catastrophe of it. In fact, you may discover that you actually have compassion for the rain. When you step into your experience, you can see that you are doing your best with what life has given you. You try less to engineer an outcome and allow yourself to join with your life rather than wish that it were different.

Admit that it is a bad day. Give in, grab the remote, open your favorite book, and park on the couch. Such a relief.

Placement

I sit down, close my eyes, and take a deep breath in. Exhale. Deep breath in. Exhale. Deep breath in. Exhale. My intention is to meditate, to keep my thoughts from drifting forward or backward. I want to stay frozen in the space between thoughts where all that exists is my breath. It would be beautiful. It would be serene. I would understand that in the nothingness I am so much bigger than my thoughts. In that single instant would stand eternity where everything is as it should be.

> When you step into your experience, you can see that you are doing your best with what life has given you. You try less to engineer an outcome and allow yourself to join with your life rather than wish that it were different.

I practice at this, and most days, I spend thirty minutes jumping from thought to thought. I make grocery lists, think I'm about to sneeze, think about today's task list, think about this book, and spend a lot of time reminding myself to go back to where I started. Deep breath in. Exhale. Each meditation session makes me keenly aware of how little time I spend in the present moment and how much effort it takes to return to the present, over and over again.

Presence is a repetitious practice. In his book *Turning the Mind into an Ally*, Sakyong Mipham talks about the "nine stages of training the mind."[26] The first four stages are about placement. Meditation is a practice of placing your mind on the moment over and over again. Placement is deliberate. It is a conscious action that takes effort. Just as when my back was having spasms in the car, I had to bring myself back to the moment over and over again. You will have to do the same. Your mind jumps to worry, bring it back. Your mind jumps to regrets, bring it back. Your mind jumps to tomorrow's medical test, bring it back. Your mind jumps to why you're sick, bring it back.

Placement is a way we exercise control in an uncontrollable situation. Being present is how we take ownership of the mind.

When Phillip and I were teaching our dog Emma to sit and stay, we would say "sit" and she would sit. Then we would say "stay" and she would pop up and trot off. We would guide her back to where we started and say "sit" again. On the "stay" command, she would pop back up. Over and over, we would guide her back and remind her to stay. We must train our minds in the same way— especially when we're working with pain and fear. Your mind will trot off years into the future, and you will have to bring it back to the truth. Again and again you will ask, "What are the facts about my situation?" and "How do I feel about those facts?"

A Conversation with Sandra Joseph, Broadway Star Staying Present with a Cranial Nerve Tumor

Sandra Joseph is staying present with a tumor on her twelfth cranial nerve. She is a singer, actress, teacher,

---

26 Sakyong Mipham, *Turning the Mind into an Ally*, (New York: Riverhead Books, 2003), 115.

and writer best known for playing the longest running Christine Daaé in *The Phantom of the Opera* on Broadway. She has been featured on *Oprah*, CNN, *The Today Show*, *The Early Show*, *Dateline*, and *The View*. Visit her at: *www.sandrajoseph.com.*

"You are no longer afraid. You have looked at the reality of what is and embraced it. With my job, for ten years, to unmask the phantom toward the end of the play, Christine learns to look at him just as he is—good, bad, and ugly—with unconditional love and acceptance. I think that is what we need to do with our lives, starting with looking in the mirror [at] who we are, our flaws and weaknesses, and the things we beat ourselves up about, and bring unconditional acceptance to ourselves. Then turn that outward, and look at the given circumstances."

Sandra's goal of unconditional acceptance became more poignant with her diagnosis, which came unexpectedly.

"I didn't even have any symptoms that led me to this diagnosis. I was diagnosed because I had another thing going on that turned out to not be a big deal at all. But while I was being tested for that, they saw on the MRI that I had this tumor in my head. Suddenly I am stuck with an awareness of something which may have been sitting there with me for years, all along; but now I have fear, which I didn't have before."

Working with that fear became a practice in presence—something she had read about from the beloved spiritual teachers Byron Katie and Eckhart Tolle. "I wish I could say that I was living in the Byron Katie–Eckhart Tolle space. I am not. I am not enlightened. I am just on the path every day like everybody else, doing the best that I can with the tools that I've learned, and obviously some days are better than others."

The teachers Sandra studies help her to see that in each moment the future is only a perception.

"If I perceive myself as someone who is sick, or someone with a tumor, or someone in danger, then I carry that weight around with me all the time. Those are the glasses through which I see the world, and suddenly everything around me becomes dark, and dangerous, and foreboding. But if I didn't know I had that tumor, and I could have gone maybe the rest of my life not knowing, I would be looking at the world through different eyes and just enjoy living my life. But I'm so grateful, I really am. I'm not grateful that I have it, but I'm grateful in a weird way that I know about it, because every challenge wakes us up."

Sandra's tumor is benign, but it is sitting on her twelfth cranial nerve, which controls the right side of her tongue, a crucial area for a woman whose career is centered on singing. As she puts it, "If they zap the tumor, it will destroy the nerve, which means I will have a speech impediment and absolutely never sing again."

A woman after my own heart, Sandra recognizes that her tumor can be used as a catalyst for personal growth. "Every painful circumstance that comes our way is a call to attention. In some ways, the negative things that come into our lives are an easier path toward presence than the day-to-day when life is cruising along going fine. I feel like one of the ways that I stay present is by acknowledging that there are challenges, by being awake and aware to the gifts that every day brings. I think my health challenges can be a path toward [spiritual] awakening."

> I'm so grateful, I really am. Because every challenge wakes us up.

Sandra's background was very different from her welcoming perspective now. She recalls, "I have about 150 aunts, uncles, cousins, and family members that still all live in the Detroit area. I grew up with these hardcore ethnic people who were very dramatic and very gloom and doom sometimes. There were a lot of funerals to go to. When you have a family of that size there are a lot of weddings, but unfortunately, also a ton of funerals. I had never really been shown any sort of hopeful response to anyone being ill. It was always catastrophizing, awfulizing, and beating of the chest."

For Sandra, the practice of being present resides in being honest with herself about what is true. I asked her how she brings herself back to the truth. Her answer is right outside her window. "I'm looking out at the snow on a tree right now, trying to love what is, as I really want it to just be spring. The tag line that I've lived by is 'living an unmasked life'; to not deny your honest feelings about anything. I think those are critical pieces of the puzzle, that you are really honest, first of all, with yourself. For example, today I'm feeling really lazy and uninspired, and that doesn't necessarily line up with how I see myself in the world and who I want to be. But that's the truth of the matter. You're going to have days like that when you're feeling unproductive, and then hopefully you can change your state and snap out of it to get done what you need to get done that day."

When Sandra finds herself lost in thoughts, worries, and assumptions, she turns to the wisdom of her body, which is always in the present moment. "Whenever I have a choice to make, when I'm trying to figure something out, a problem I'm struggling with, I try to listen to my body and breathe into the yes and no to see how my body feels. Some people feel it in their stomach, or in their chest. I think so many women try to pretend. They try to put on the mask [and think,] 'I've got it all under control. Everything is great. I'm superwoman!' And really, we're exhausting ourselves. I'm a big fan of keeping it real with yourself and with other people."

Sandra has come to a peaceful relationship with her tumor. "It is just my pal. We are hanging out on this ride together. I really do feel that way about it. I don't fear it. I don't hate it. I fully embrace it as a part of me that I'm just going to groove with for the rest of time. I don't personally believe that it's going to disappear." Sandra monitors the tumor through annual MRIs. So far, it is still there but unchanged. "If the time comes that it does change, I believe that I would have what it takes to get through that experience, whatever that means."

Going for her annual MRI gives Sandra a chance to practice working with fear. "I've not had one single MRI when I didn't burst into tears on the table because it's just freaky. It scares me every time. Even though I try to practice everything I know: meditate before, listen to tapes, CDs, the whole thing. I still have a really emotional, visceral response when they clamp my head down. They put you in this Freddy Krueger mask. You're lying there, and you can't move. For me, because of my tumor, I can't swallow, and it takes about forty-five minutes. Trying to lie perfectly still and not swallow for forty-five minutes is a challenge. I always have a bit of a meltdown. I try to just tell myself that whatever the outcome is, I will have the skills and the support system to deal with it and be OK. I have friends and family who will be there for me. I can rely on my own core inner strength."

Sandra intimately knows that strength from grieving the loss of her father. "My dad was like my heart. We were extremely close. He was my biggest fan and supporter. He died suddenly of a heart attack in 2007, and I was so anguished by that loss. I had feared it all my life. All my life I thought, 'Oh my God! When my dad goes, I'm just not going to want to go on.' In the midst of that loss I was surrounded by compassion, a compassionate presence that felt like it was carrying me along through the days, and I felt so supported. The word people would use for it is grace, and I just believe that whatever happens with this tumor, or whatever life brings, I believe in the power of grace to carry me through."

In a seminar with Eckhart Tolle at the Omega Institute right after September 11th, Sandra had a profound experience of presence. As she and the other students were grieving along with the country, she could see that she was bigger, separate from her emotions. She was the witness to the emotion. "There is a beautiful separation that occurs between my feelings and the witness [to those feelings]. As you fully experience your emotions, there is a split where you realize, 'I am not my emotions. My emotions are coming through me, but the pain that I'm feeling right now, or the fear, or whatever the emotion is, is not who I am.' There's a separation. It's like you're watching yourself cry, in a weird way. Bringing that kind of compassionate presence to our experience in the moment that we're experiencing it will carry us through.

"I remember being on the bathroom floor at four o'clock in the morning after my father died and sobbing, and sobbing, and sobbing. The tiles under my eyes were a blur, but I remember that experience of being a witness, that there was some part of me watching me on the bathroom floor. So that it [the grief] didn't consume me entirely, that sadness and the anguish didn't swallow me up. There's something beyond. That's where my faith comes in. It really has been my experience that the hard times, the most painful things I've gone through, are the things that have given me a solid sense of self that I've always lacked. Now, having lived through some really painful challenges, I feel like I've finally found my footing and found my center."

Sandra is working on her first book. She continues to teach, perform, and live an unmasked life as she steps toward the painful stuff to live fully into who she is. Sandra reminds us, "It really always comes back to presence."

HEALTH TIPS

- Notice which thoughts create stress.

- To come back to the present moment, ask: "What are the facts of my situation?" and "How do I feel about those facts?"

- Take advantage of good days by doing things you enjoy.

- Honor bad days by becoming present and feeling how you feel without judging yourself for it.

- Presence is a practice, something you do over and over again.

CHAPTER 9

Cultivate Discipline

I am not one of those people who sets a goal and effortlessly skips to its completion. I have backslides, internal "do I have to?" conversations, and years of starting and stopping worthy pursuits.

Just as spring was fading into summer a few years back, I joined an accountability group. Each morning, at 5:00 A.M. no less, I would lurch out of bed, let the dogs out, and plop onto the couch to call in with the other participants to see if we were accomplishing what we set out to. I was in full goal mode, attempting to eat healthier, exercise, meditate, read more, journal, and the list went on and on. I was making progress with some and feeling guilty about others. As summer heated up, I was growing weary of the struggle to hold myself accountable.

That August, Phillip and I were going to leave Portland and return to California for a job opportunity. From having made these moves before, I knew that setting up house in a new state can be daunting. When I set my goals for the month of the move, I got a brilliant idea: my only goal during August was to be kind to myself. That's it. Just kind, not forced to eat spinach, sit in silence, or get twisted in yoga postures. My 5:00 A.M. comrades agreed; my idea was genius. Here is how the month of our move went down.

Scene 1

Thought: I should meditate.

Action: No meditation. (I was being "kind" to myself and didn't feel like it.)

Thought: You really should have meditated.

Response: I am being "kind" this month—let it go.

Result: Fits of feeling overwhelmed and stressed-out crying from the move.

Scene 2

Thought: You shouldn't eat that third slice of pizza and finish it off with ice cream.

Action: Scarf down third slice like I'm never going to eat again and drown my guilt in ice cream. (I was being "kind" and allowing myself treats.)

Thought: You definitely should not have eaten that.

Response: Be quiet me! I am being *kiiiiiiinnnd* this month.

Result: No action due to low energy. Lie on the couch.

My "month of kindness" was turning me into a mess. I was on edge, tired, overwhelmed, and as Phillip can attest to, very easily upset.

Even though I have backslides, internal "Do I have to?" conversations, and years of starting and stopping worthy pursuits, I have realized that it is the discipline to start each day with fresh commitment that is the true kindness.

The Pitfall

Humans come from a long line of innovators. Millennia ago, we realized that it is hard work to hunt and gather. We started looking for high calorie foods that could be obtained in the quickest way possible. In time, we grew crops and herded animals so that our hunting and gathering could happen at our doorstep. This mindset took us far. Very, very far. Through the industrial revolution to the Internet. Medicine, once a crude practice of leaches and lobotomies, has made exponential strides to create a plethora of cure-all pills. The search for a quick fix has been baked into our DNA. We've gotten used to the effortless solution.

Illness doesn't always have a quick fix, and that can be baffling. It goes against what we've gotten used to. That doesn't mean we don't still try to find it. The $20 billion dollar weight loss industry is a testament to our searching.[27] Once we find what we think will be the holy grail of a cure, we try it, lose interest, declare that it didn't work, and move on to the next fad. You've got the ThighMaster stuffed under your bed, Chinese herbs in your medicine cabinet, and you've cleaned out the pantry with declaration of a reformed diet (several times). You find yourself adding to your bookshelf and credit card debt with promises that don't keep. Unfortunately, so, so very unfortunately, there isn't always a magic pill. The magic you're searching for comes from the promises you keep to yourself.

When you declare that "tomorrow I will stop eating sugar" and find that by 10:00 A.M. the next day you've got your hand on a doughnut because, "well, it's a special

---

27 ABC News Staff, "100 Million Dieters, $20 Billion: The Weight Loss Industry by the Numbers," ABC 20-20 (May, 2012). *abcnews.go.com.*

occasion," you dent your self-confidence. If a friend promises to visit you on Tuesday and doesn't, then promises to visit on Thursday and doesn't, then says she'll come Saturday and doesn't, do you trust her anymore? Heck no. You erode your own trust in the same way. Each broken promise makes it harder to believe in yourself and your ability to do what you say you will.

Changing a habit is hard. It is one of the hardest things you will tackle in your life. Marketers love to make us think that change is easy. They use words like: simple, immediate, effective, effortless, instant. Our expectations are set up for easy. Yet, expecting things to be easy only makes them harder. Expectation is the pitfall. Whatever it is that is going to help your health, I can tell you it will be work. Lots of work. Work on the external stuff and work on the internal stuff. Work that you are absolutely capable of doing, but work nonetheless.

> Our expectations are set up for easy. Yet, expecting things to be easy only makes them harder.

The Paradox

Jane Fonda made an appearance on *Anderson Cooper* and revealed that she does not like to work out. Jane Fonda, the legwarmer fitness guru of the 1980s, does not like to work out! I was floored. She doesn't wake up in the morning revved to get up and into the gym, but she does it anyway. She works out each day because she feels better after it's over. That's the key.

There is a paradox of coping with an illness that each woman faces: we don't feel like doing what will help us to feel better.

I never feel like taking my medications. I don't jump for joy at eating kale and brown rice for dinner. I do those things because I know that although I don't feel like doing them in the moment, I will feel better thirty minutes, an hour, two hours, two years down the road because I did them. It is hard to make the right choice for our future self because she isn't here with us today. The self we've got today wants to stay in bed and skip the workout. She is the one who wants the double hot fudge sundae. Our desire for immediate gratification is putting us through all sorts of crap.

At sixteen, when I was getting frequent kidney infections, I was prescribed a daily low-dose antibiotic to prevent urinary tract infections, which were quickly becoming kidney infections due to my kidney reflux. If I missed one pill, just one, I would have a kidney infection the next day. I didn't have a great method for being disciplined about remembering to take my medication and as a result did more damage to my kidney.

Now I have more medications and a new routine that ensures I swallow what I've been prescribed. Each Sunday night I ritually fill my pill sorters. I've got one for the morning and one for the evening. I think about it once during the week and swallow a handful twice a day without giving it a second thought. Less than 50 percent of all prescribed medication is actually taken by the patient it is prescribed for.[28] Because women forget, or want to avoid their diagnosis all together, they set themselves up for pain or other more serious health crises.

When you are prescribed a medication, make sure you know what it is for, the side effects, and the instructions for taking it. In your doctor's office is the place to discuss the pros and cons of being on a medication.

---

28 Jeffrey Boyd, *Being Sick Well: Joyful Living Despite Chronic Illness* (Michigan: Baker Books, 2005), 16.

If you know that you will not fill or take a medication your doctor thinks you are taking, tell her. Your doctor needs to know what you are, or are not, doing at home so that she can help you manage your health. If your doctor is unwilling to work with you to find a medication or alternative treatment that you are comfortable with, seek out a new doctor. If you begin taking a medication and notice side effects that are concerning, contact your doctor to let her know what is going on. If you agree that you should be taking what you're prescribed, take it. Set timers, get pill sorters, put the pill bottles on your nightstand, do what you need to do to remember to take your meds.

Feelings are strong and persuasive. Feelings want you to fit in by eating cake with everyone else, and they demand the comfort of a couch instead of the confining rubber of tennis shoes. Especially when you don't feel well or you're stressed, you want to soothe yourself and save your energy. However, greasy food and a sedentary lifestyle provide little benefit when you're trying to regain your health.

Discipline is the move from short- to long-term thinking. Let your twenty-twenty hindsight be the decision maker. When you're beginning to have an internal conversation that starts with "I should," as in "I should take a walk," or "I should take my supplements," ask yourself how you will feel after accomplishing the end of that sentence. If the answer is great, energetic, or proud, do it now. Get it over with so you can get to the good feelings that come from putting in the effort.

> You know what you've got to do. Procrastinating just prolongs the dread that it's coming. Get in. Get it done.

Some healthy behaviors may not have an immediate, or immediately desirable, benefit. Going to dialysis, chemotherapy, physical therapy, taking your medication, and a host of other treatments can be time-consuming, annoying, or make you feel miserable. Treatments are also reminders that you need treatment, which can trigger pesky worries and foggy gloom. Long-term thinking in this case is to focus on the feeling of relief that you're getting it over with. Your treatment decision has been made. You know what you've got to do. Procrastinating just prolongs the dread that it's coming. Get in. Get it done.

The life coach and radio host Mel Robbins is a pioneer for forcing ourselves to do what will help us accomplish our goals. She says that the force needed to do something you don't feel like doing is the same force it takes to get out of a warm bed and into a cold room when your alarm goes off.[29] The first cold steps on your way to the bathroom are never pleasant, but once you've peed, things seem better. Once you've had your tea and washed your face, you're feeling awake, and once you're into your day, you are glad you got up early. It is that way with new habits. Overcoming the paradox that will keep you in your pj's eating ice cream for dinner takes force, lots and lots of force.

Standards

There are certain standards that most people hold themselves accountable to. We are so regimented about these that we hardly consider not doing them. Rather than let fuzz grow on your teeth or have them rot out of your head you brush them; you shower so that you'll be welcome in public places; and you live in a place that has walls and a roof because the rain is cold. There are hundreds of these small standards that you keep because the consequences of not doing them are unpleasant at best and dire at worst.

---

29 Mel Robbins, "How to Stop Screwing Yourself." Video, June, 2011. *www.youtube.com.*

Did you ever think that you don't have to keep to your standards? There are people who choose to be homeless or that don't practice regular hygiene. One episode of *Hoarding: Buried Alive* will chillingly demonstrate that standards are a thing of personal preference. Since I assume you aren't the woman who throws her used diabetes injection needles on the trash heap in her living room, you've got the basics of standards down. You are an expert at deciding what your standards are and keeping them.

Your body is asking you to raise your standards to a level that supports your whole health: mind, body, and spirit. There are new things that your doctors and your intuition are asking you to incorporate into your routine. This is the time to go back to your research in chapter 7 and back to your doctor's instructions to determine what your new standards are.

Some of your standards will be must-dos. Others will fall into the category of "makes me happy/reduces stress." Standards are different for everyone, and yours will be unique to your diagnosis.

The only thing about standards is they must be absolute; when we give ourselves wiggle room, we tend to wiggle right out. Conversely, deciding that your standards are nonnegotiable gets them done. No muss, and definitely no fuss. Just like brushing your teeth each and every day.

MY STANDARDS

Make a list of everything that you are going to hold yourself accountable for. Start with what you must do to maintain your health. Next, think about the best ways to reduce stress. Follow with those things that make you proud of who you are, the ones that honor your family and your planet.

Self-help superhero Tony Robbins has said that raising his standards is the biggest positive change he made in his life. Defining his standards helped him become the übermotivator he is today.

When I took the time to list my standards, I saw myself in a new light. I saw the person I wanted to become and knew I could start being. Having something written helped guide my behaviors. Here are some of my standards:

- Take medications and supplements in the morning and evening.

- Check blood pressure daily.

- Exercise four times per week.

- Follow a vegan diet.

- Include a fruit or vegetable with each meal.

- Don't overeat.

- Devote thirty minutes to spiritual practice five times per week.

- Talk positively about others.

- Respect myself, including what I say about me.

- Make a prioritized list of tasks to do each day.

- No dishes in the sink or laundry on the floor, and make the bed.

Is my list perfect? No. Could I do better? Yes. At this time, the items above are what I am willing to commit to. Commitment is vital. Without it, your standards will only be ways to whip up some guilt. If you know that you're not going to do yoga every day, then don't list it. List something that you are likely to do that might lead to yoga, such as five minutes of daily stretching.

It is important that your standards are specific. If they aren't, you won't know how to implement them, and you'll be back to wiggling out of them. A few times over the years I have given up sugar. If I say I'm going to eat less sugar or even "only have sugar on special occasions," then suddenly the fact that the mail came is cause to bake some cookies. For me, "less sugar" has to be "no sugar." The more specific your standards, the easier they are to implement.

SCHEDULING STANDARDS

For each standard you plan to implement, choose a day and time that you will complete the task.

Once your standards are listed, revamp your daily schedule to include them. For each standard you've written in your journal, ask "when will I do this?" From those answers, write out a weekly schedule that gives specific times for your standards. Based on my list above, my schedule looks like this:

Daily

- Medications: 7:30 A.M. and 9:30 P.M.
- Make the bed/straighten up: 8:00 A.M.
- Check blood pressure: 9:00 A.M.
- Create tomorrow's task list: 6:00 P.M.

Monday Through Friday

- Spiritual Practice: 8:30 A.M.

Monday, Wednesday, Thursday and Saturday

- Work out: 6:15 A.M. (8:15 on Saturday)

Sunday

- Create grocery list and shop

Put this schedule into Outlook, your smartphone, your calendar, anywhere that will remind you of what you said you were going to do. If your standards involve taking medications, dialysis, checking insulin, or other medical procedures, set an alarm on your phone. You'll forget otherwise—trust me.

Your motivation to step up your game got huge with your diagnosis. If not now, when? If not for your health, then for what?

Start Small

When I set my summertime goal of trying one new thing each week (see chapter 3), I went to the Ananda Portland meditation center to participate in an hour-long 6:00 A.M. meditation session. Up to that point, I had been a sporadic meditator who, at most, practiced for thirty minutes. I spent most of the hour meditating on the thought, "Is this over yet?" I never went back to the center and had to ease back into meditating after a few months break. Too much too fast will have you napping through your commitment to exercise.

> Too much too fast will have you napping through your commitment to exercise.

BJ Fogg, PhD, a professor at Stanford University, did an at-home experiment related to his work as a behavior researcher. He wanted to change his behavior; specifically, he wanted to join the ranks of daily teeth flossers. Based on his research in the lab, he knew that behavior changes are best accomplished when you start small; hence, he started with the goal of flossing one tooth.[30] If he could do that, then he could declare his mission

---

30 BJ Fogg, PhD. Interview by Ramit Sethi. "Hustle Your Way to the Top. I Will Teach You to Be Rich," 2011. *www.iwillteachyoutoberich.com*.

accomplished for the day. What happens? You floss one tooth and keep going until you have a sparkling smile.

START SMALL

What small steps will you take to implement each of your new standards?

The same goes for implementing your standards. Start small. Don't try to become a vegan marathon runner all in one fell swoop. The first step might be to give up beef and walk fifteen minutes each day. Turn back to the page in your journal with your standards. What is reasonable to start with? Pick one or two standards to focus on now. If your goal is to meditate for thirty minutes each day, start with ten minutes, or even five minutes, four times a week. If you want to work out for an hour, begin with just fifteen sit-ups and five pushups each day. Instead of going cold turkey on the coffee, switch to black tea. Once you see some results from your first wave of implementation, your motivation will be stronger to keep going. Of course, be sure to check with your health care provider before implementing any dietary changes or exercise routines.

Our behavior largely determines our attitude.

You can't think your way into healthy behaviors. It would be lovely if merely having the right attitude could lead to the right actions. But, alas, research shows that it is the other way around. Our behavior largely determines our attitude.[31] Accomplishing your morning workout and seeing your muscles build makes you feel energized and proud. You can drive to the gym as grumpy as you want, but after a few months there, you will find your attitude about your body and the gym shifting.

---

31 Ibid.

Twenty-One-Day Bologna

Have you ever heard that it takes three weeks to establish a new habit? That's simply not true. Maybe it is true in the laboratory with research participants, but out here in the land of temptation and warm beds, it is easy to break a habit you've been doing consistently for three weeks. Go on vacation, get sick, stay up late, have a headache, forget or not be in the mood, and the habit is long gone.

One year my New Year's resolution was to try an exercise I had adapted from the book *You Already Know What to Do* by Sharon Franquemont.[32] I wrote myself a letter about all that I had accomplished and read it into a tape recorder. Each morning, I moved from the bed to the couch and listened to my recording. I did this each morning for thirty mornings, and I had great results. My confidence was booming. I had more energy and was making strides in my business. On the thirty-first morning, I stopped. I tried to start up a few times after that and would listen to various affirmations sporadically, but I never repeated the exercise that was supposed to be an ingrained habit after not three but four full weeks.

> When you are coping with illness, *chronic resilience* is the mantra. You've got to find the persistence to keep going after the third, fourth, and fortieth week of doing what you know is best for you.

When you are coping with illness, *chronic resilience* is the mantra. You've got to find the persistence to keep going after the third, fourth, and fortieth week of doing what you know is best for you. There is no secret. Your discipline is what makes the difference. Discipline for the long haul. Discipline when you plateau. Discipline

---

32 Sharon Franquemont, *You Already Know What to Do*. New York: Jeremy P. Tarcher/Putnam, 1999), 60–61.

when the last thing you want to do is put your butt on the meditation cushion. Discipline when you are being pulled in eight different directions. Discipline when your to-do list is long. Discipline when you feel well, and discipline when you don't.

If-Then Planning

Try as you might, various things *will* distract you from your standards. You will go on vacation, and once home, your 6:00 A.M. alarm will seem harshly cruel. Most people hit snooze and don't attempt to exercise again until the ball drops at midnight. There is another approach. Motivation researchers Gabriele Oettingen and Peter Gollwitzer have seen self-discipline increase with use of a technique called if-then planning.[33] Before you leave your house to vacation on the warm beaches of Hawaii, think about how you will get back on track once you're home. For example, *if* you feel tired, *then* you will splash cold water on your face. *If* you sleep through your alarm, *then* you will work out at lunch. *If* it is hard to get out of bed, *then* you will put your alarm across the room. Decide on what your approach will be and mentally rehearse your if-then scenario a few times before you have to get up again. This technique can be applied to all sorts of conundrums: birthday cake at work, getting a cold, staying up too late, forgetting to go to yoga, getting busy at work, etc.

> Before you leave your home to vacation on the warm beaches of Hawaii, think about how you will get back on track once you're home.

------

33   Paul M. Gollwitzer and Gabriele Oettingen, "The Role of Goal Setting and Goal Striving in Medical Adherence" In *Medical Adherence and Aging. Social and Cognitive Perspectives*, D. C. Park and L. L. Liu (eds.), Washington, DC: American Psychological Association, 2007, 23–47.

Our best intentions don't have to be our forgotten intentions because something comes up. Find your chronic resilience and get back to it.

Take Measurements

Changes can be subtle. Measuring the success of your standards will make small improvements more obvious. Here are some ways to measure your successes:

- Assess your pain daily using a 1 (zilch) to 10 (knock me out now) pain scale.

- Assess your level of stress daily using a 1 (in bliss) to 10 (pulling my hair out) scale.

- Assess your energy level daily on a 1 (can't keep my eyes open) to 10 (want to bound up a mountain) scale.

- Chart the number of inches you've lost.

- Chart the number of pounds you've lost.

- Monitor your blood pressure. Drug stores carry monitors for at-home use.

- Record how often you have arguments with family.

- Keep track of how many times you say something you didn't mean to.

- Track your trips to, or hours spent in, the little girls' room. (Yeah, you know what I'm taking about.)

- Chart your minutes of free time.

- Notice the number of pages you've written in your journal.

- Record your daily servings of fruits and veggies.

- Notice how many hours of TV you've watched.

- Record how many minutes you've spent in meditation.

Discipline isn't the practice of forcing yourself to do things that don't work. If one of your standards is no longer working, drop it.

Accountability

If you are not naturally gifted at discipline, then you are going to need someone to hold you accountable to your standards. As hard as most women are on ourselves, we have become experts at finding inventive excuses for not meeting our goals. We end up mentally ignoring the slip-up, or drowning in guilt for letting another weekend go by without exercising.

We want to please others and won't do for ourselves what we are quick to do for someone else. It is how we're built. Though I may be inconsistent about some habits, I am 100 percent regimented when it comes to announcing my plans. I need my husband, friends, and family to know what I'm up to so that I actually do it. If I am struggling with something big, I get professional help. A life coach is great at asking you if you did what you said you were going to do. You could find a trainer or join a class. Knowing that your neighbor is waiting for you to join her on a walk will surely get you out of bed.

If you are focused on diet, a nutritionist can steer you in the right direction. There are also lots of diet programs and websites that provide support and regular check-ins. Another way to focus on diet is to find a group of likeminded women who take turns hosting a potluck dinner party where you share favorite healthy dishes.

For pursuits of the spiritual nature, join religious study groups at your church or synagogue. There are also lots of meditation groups and classes where you can meet other people who share your goals.

In chapter 2, we spent some time determining what your values are. Like goals, your standards are the ways that you live your values. They are the motivation behind staying the course. Did you list family or love as one of your values? The discipline to take care of your health is a way to honor the people you love. Becoming healthier and less stressed opens up your capacity for love. Being on edge because you're trying to do it all is not being the heroine. The heroine is the woman who puts her standards at the top of her list. She knows that if she takes a walk in the morning, takes time to cook and eat nutritiously, and spends thirty minutes in prayer she will be more attentive and able to manage the stresses that come up during the day. Making your standards a priority is not selfish; it is the way you protect your health and energy to better provide for your loved ones.

Being on edge because you're trying to do it all is not being the heroine. The heroine is the woman who puts her standards at the top of her list.

Forgiveness

I mess up. I have a great list of standards, and I still miss a few from time to time. A rainy morning and I'll sleep through my workout. I meditate consistently for weeks and then skip a few days. These things happen. I am not perfect yet. You are not perfect yet. We are still human. Forgiveness is a key ingredient in discipline. If each slip up causes you to determine that you have no willpower and that you will never accomplish your goal, you will have a tough road ahead. It is important to feel like we can do what we say we are going to. If each missed workout or French fry order adds to the evidence that you are unable to trust yourself, you erode your belief that you can stick to your standards.

However, a skipped workout met with forgiveness becomes a onetime thing. You know that you will go at it again tomorrow. There is no shame in being human. We have failures, we have challenges; they don't make us bad people. The failures and challenges are why we need to be chronically resilient. Start each day with an intention to be disciplined. Take it one action and decision at a time. If old habits take over and you find yourself with a pint of Cherry Garcia, forgive yourself and have an apple tomorrow.

A Conversation with Mari Ruddy, Diabetic, Two-Time Breast Cancer Survivor, and Founder of TeamWILD

Mari Ruddy is a two-time breast cancer survivor focused on athletics while managing type 1 diabetes. She is the founder and director of TeamWILD, which provides resources and inspiration for people with diabetes to become athletes. Visit her at: *www.teamwildathletics.com.*

"I had been teaching student leadership, so I knew a lot about how to manage a project, and I made my health a project. That was the beginning of my athletic journey, and it was extremely difficult. I have low blood pressure, so when I would exercise, I wouldn't be able to tell the difference between low blood sugar, low blood pressure, and physical exertion."

Diabetes runs in Mari's family. She was diagnosed at sixteen. After seeing her father have some scary episodes due to low blood sugar, Mari subconsciously ran her blood sugars high to avoid what she had witnessed with her father. At age thirty, her hemoglobin A1c [a measure of blood sugar] was dangerously high. That was her wakeup call to become disciplined about her health. It also sparked a passion for fitness that would transform Mari's life.

After three years of research, working with a trainer, and religiously checking her blood sugar during exercise, Mari gained confidence in her athletic abilities—enough to attempt a four-hundred-mile bike ride across the state of Colorado. "When I decided that I wanted to do my first bicycle ride, my relationship with diabetes dramatically changed, and my relationship with how I ate changed because I wanted to perform on that ride. I was bound and determined to make it all four hundred miles riding my bike the entire time. For the preceding five or six months that I was training, I would open my refrigerator and make a choice about what I was going to eat based on if it was going to help me get across the state of Colorado: 'If I eat chocolate cake right now, is that the best choice?' It was less about diabetes than about my goal of performance. That mindset continues to be my number one motivator."

Mari assembled a team to make sure her ride was safe and successful. "I had an endocrinologist and a cycling coach who supported me through the training process. I had them talk to each other about me. I had the cycling coach read several books about diabetes, fitness, and exercise, and I had the endocrinologist read about cycling. I encouraged each of them to go outside their profession to be able to support me. Then I did the ride and it was very successful."

However, her body was slow to recover afterward. "They could not figure out what was wrong with me. They did all these tests and nothing was conclusive. The ride was in June of 2004, then in October 2004, I found the lump in my breast. Yes, I had breast cancer."

Cancer treatments are rough, and Mari's body reacted harshly to the hormone therapy prescribed. She ended up taking a three-month leave of absence from her work to fully recover. Through grief therapy and the support of her friends and family, she eventually got back to life as usual.

Then, in July 2010, she again found that she wasn't recovering, this time from a marathon. "I found another lump in the same breast, so I went in." It was a second breast cancer. "I had a mastectomy. It hadn't spread anywhere else in my body. They determined that it was a second primary cancer, which means that it was not a recurrence, which was odd. It was as if my body had started over from zero, growing another cancer as if I had never had cancer before."

Throughout Mari's life she has had pivotal moments. At these times, she reassesses and redoubles her commitment. These moments "were not revelations, per se; they were just very sure awarenesses and wisdom that I knew were true for me. The element of truth is what would sustain me." After her mastectomy, Mari needed to decide if she was going to try hormone therapy once more to supplement her latest cancer treatment. She decided to take a different approach.

"I chose not to do any of the drugs that they wanted me to do because the drugs are really just an insurance policy. There's no guarantee that I wouldn't grow cancer a third time, and the quality of my life would have been dramatically impacted because the drugs are so potent. I would have instantly felt like I was ninety-five years old. My joints would ache, my muscles would hurt twenty-four hours a day, my eyes would be dry all the time, and I would have zero sex drive. [I thought,] I'd rather live ten years feeling fantastic, instead of thirty years feeling like shit. I did what most people with cancer do not do: I became a pretty strict vegan. I worked on my stress levels every day. I worked on having a meditation practice, and I really looked at what I was doing with my life and what has deep meaning for me. Because if I only get ten or twenty years, how do I want to spend that time?"

The mindset for making such disciplined and dramatic changes was ingrained in Mari. It is the spirit of TeamWILD Athletics, a resource for people with diabetes wanting to maintain an active lifestyle. "At TeamWILD, we teach people with diabetes how to see themselves as athletes first and people who have a health condition second. The idea is that athletes take really good care of their bodies. Athletes have a physical goal that's about performance and celebration. Instead of being motivated to exercise because you have to, because the doctor told you to, I would much rather people start with changing their minds. Decide that you're an athlete first, all by itself. Don't worry about all the reasons you can't be an athlete; don't worry about all the reasons someone told you that you should not be an athlete: you're not fast enough, you're not coordinated enough, you're not gifted enough. Then start acting like an athlete who has whatever [disease] you have.

"[For example,] you're an athlete, and now you have diabetes. How are you going to take care of your diabetes from the lens of being an athlete? Well, you're going to find out how insulin works in your body because you've got to know how your insulin works to be a better athlete. You've got to train because all athletes train. You're not just going to go exercise at the gym; you're going to have a plan because you're going to perform at an event. That's what athletes do.

"What event do you want to train for, and what kind of plan do you need for your particular challenges? Find a coach who will work with you, not because you have diabetes, but because they're a coach who's going to work with you to get you to your event with your particular challenges. Because that's what good coaches do."

Given Mari's dynamic view of her health and her relationship to her body, I asked for her top three tips to keep health goals in view. "The number one thing is to keep the goal in front of you. Periodically ask, 'What is my goal?' and make it as specific as possible. Choose one thing to focus on at a time. It's much easier to maintain discipline and maintain focus if you know what it is that you're focusing on, and why it matters to you. That's the first thing.

"The second thing is, who's on your team? Every one of us deserves to have tools and people that are part of our individual team. Assess whoever's on your team. Are they the right people? Do periodic evaluations of who's helping you and who's hurting you. Helping you might not mean that they're coddling you, but that they're pushing you to new heights, helping you view your blind spots, as well as supporting you.

"The third key thing that I always emphasize with everybody is to have a good time with it. So much of life is heavy, and when you have a chronic thing, that can really wear you down. [Ask yourself] 'Am I having a good time? Am I laughing?'"

This third key is something Mari actively works on. After pushing herself to grow TeamWILD, she has realized that she needs more pivotal moments, more quiet spaces to listen to where life is leading her. "Essentially, for the last year and a half, I've worked almost every single day, from a minimum of six hours a day, and often more like ten hours a day. Seven days a week." Her new discipline is to insert moments of meditation and relaxation into days that only include three hours of work with lots of time to focus on her health. To achieve this goal, she has turned to her tried and true methods of training for an event. "One of the things that's kind of cool that I've done the last few days, and I do every time I train for a race, is the month and week before a race I write down my daily schedule. I write down what time I'm going to go to bed. I write down what time I'm going to wake up. I write down what time I'm going to turn off all of my electronics before I go to bed. I write down what time I'm going to eat, and what sorts of foods. I write down when I'm going to meditate, and I write down my work hours."

For Mari, discipline includes leaving room to sway from her plan. Getting off track and back on is all part of the athlete mindset. "There's a concept in endurance athletics that's called 'periodization.'" She says that when athletes train, they divide time into cycles of activity and rest. "In periodization, you focus on different things at different times . . . within a week, you always have a rest day; within a month, you have a rest week; and within a season, you have rest phases. Where you become faster or stronger is not actually when you work out. It's when you rest. That's when your muscles grow and the body adapts. It's in the repair and recovery phase that you become a better athlete.

"In the diabetes component of our program we teach that you cannot keep yourself to the same high expectations of performance when it comes to managing your diabetes every single day. You have to take a break. Knowing that up front is so relieving. On vacation, do a little more guessing than you normally would, test your blood sugar a little bit less, give yourself permission to take a rest and take a break. When you come back from your vacation, sit down and ask, where am I now? What am I going to do? And how can I recommit myself? and understand that's a behavior of a very high level athlete.

"The other thing I'm a huge fan of is the 80-20 rule—or, if you're on a weight loss plan and your health is even more precarious, the 90-10 rule: 10 percent of the time you eat for your soul, and 90 percent of the time you eat for your health. Soul food might be chocolate, or whatever it is that you need for your soul. You can't be so strict all the time."

Mari continues to feed her soul by being disciplined enough to meditate, eat a plant-based diet, and see herself as an athlete first and a diabetic and cancer survivor second. That is what takes her performance to a whole new level.

HEALTH TIPS

- Let go of the search for a quick fix. Know that the magic lies in your discipline.

- Do what helps your body even when you don't feel like it.

- Make a list of your standards and create a schedule to keep them.

- Find an accountability partner.

- Forgive yourself for slip-ups. You'll try again tomorrow.

CHAPTER 10

Find Gratitude

"If I were your mother or your sister, I would beg you not to get pregnant." The room stood still. My head nodded in understanding, but I was not controlling its up-down motion. Everything felt oddly separate from me. Like I was watching my life on a stage, sitting in a dark auditorium where the lights of the OB-GYN clinic lit up a play.

I politely nodded through the rest of the appointment, but by the time we made it to the elevator, things were sinking in. I turned to Phillip and burst into tears. People crowded around us waiting for the same ding that meant we could all get out of this place. I'm sure they were staring, but the tears didn't care.

We had only been married for eight months at that time and were living in Colorado. It was an unusual day in Denver. A wayward tornado had descended onto the city, and as Phillip and I stepped through the clinic's sliding glass door and onto the sidewalk, the tornado siren began blaring. We paused, not wanting to go back inside and at the same time unsure if we should ignore the warning and take refuge in the car. We chose the car. It was too impossible to head back into a place that had just rejected my ability to become pregnant.

We ended up at the OB-GYN clinic because my doctor had recommended we see a high-risk OB-GYN specialist. We were a young married couple and would need to know the risks of managing a pregnancy with kidney disease. I expected a quick check-in and leaving with a pamphlet titled "Kidney Disease, Pregnancy, and You." Instead I got something that completely changed my life.

We weren't even trying to get pregnant. I was on a "five-year plan" for kids. I fully expected that five years after we had been married we would start a family the traditional way. Get pregnant. Have a baby shower. Read and play Mozart to my big pregnant belly as we dreamt about the day our child would be elected president.

As we drove away from the clinic, I began to process what I had just heard. The doctor told us that my kidney was an issue—a big issue. Getting pregnant would give me a 30 percent chance of needing a transplant by the end of the pregnancy or cause my blood pressure to soar dangerously high (preeclampsia) too early for a baby to be born safely. I tried to weigh the odds of myself and a child making it through a nine-month pregnancy safely, but nothing was adding up. Around the same time, we also found out that the physical abnormalities of my uterus would restrict a child's growth; plus the genetic verdict is still out on the possibility that I could pass VACTERL on to a child. The odds were quickly stacking against me.

That day at the clinic also happened to be seven months into one of my closet friend's first pregnancies. I didn't tell her the news. I wanted to share in her joys without having them filtered for my feelings. She would call and we would excitedly talk about how she was decorating the nursery and shopping for the latest in maternity wear. I would hang up and cry, sunken into my chair, blurrily staring into the dark. For four months, I grieved the loss of my fertility. I indulged my fantasies of what could have been and worked through boxes and boxes of tissues as I saw them fade from my mind. It was the best thing I could have done.

Letting Go

My neighbors have beautiful lawns: weed-free, perfectly edged, and highlighted by bright azaleas, poppies, and daffodils. Their grass is greener than mine. It is hard to be grateful when their grass is greener. The comparison dampens my appreciation for our trees and roses. It stops me from seeing that our yard is lovely too.

The hardest part of dealing with an illness is letting go of expectations. Whether we want to admit it or not, we love to paint wonderful pictures of how things are supposed to be. There is a certain path that life takes for most people, and we feel that we have the birthright to follow the same path. Illness can change everything. Family plans change, vacation plans disappear, the energy to be as productive as you once were fades along with your memory and focus. Even though the domain of illness is in the body, it reaches out to touch every area of life.

> Gratitude can coexist with illness, but only after space is made for it. That space comes from letting go.

It is natural to see your attention turn to what you must let go of when you get a diagnosis or new symptoms show up. Don't suppress this. Lean into it. Feel it. Grieve it. Allow your loss to have a voice.

Jumping from sick straight to being grateful denies your innate humanness. This type of gratitude feels forced. On the surface. Unable to sink in. As you think, "I am grateful for the health I still have," it is quickly countered with lists of what you no longer have. Gratitude can coexist with illness, but only after space is made for it. That space comes from letting go.

Opening

One evening in late September, four months after the bad news, Phillip and I were channel surfing and came to the program *Adoption Stories* on The Learning Channel. We watched as a mother traveled to Russia to adopt a one-year-old bright-eyed baby girl. I can still picture her first sweet, squishy hug with her forever mom. When the program ended, we talked about what having a child meant in our lives. For us, was it about DNA or about love? In that moment, we both realized that we had a deep-seated passion for adoption, something we never would have discovered had we not closed the door on pregnancy. From my grief, gratitude arrived.

Expectations can get in the way of opening up to life. They can cloud opportunities and blessings that already surround you. When your story about what life is "supposed" to look like falls away, when you accept your illness without judgment, then gratitude naturally shows up.

It can be scary to let things be what they are without a plan of how to fix it to be what you want. On the other hand, it can also be liberating. As you've seen in each chapter, there are a lot of things you can control; but even with all that, you can't control everything. I get tired of trying to control what isn't mine to control. It can be exhausting to plan life out and lose your plan again and again. It is relieving to turn control over and open up to where you are being led.

I opened chapter 1 with an analogy of being cast into the sea. With each wave, you kick and tread to find the shore. But what if you learned to let the shore go? What if you learned to ride the swells and swim through the waves? You could be in the water without feeling lost. You could notice the blessing that the sea is. You could be grateful.

What Is Gratitude?

Gratitude is a feeling. It is not an intellectual exercise. It is not a list that you make, or an obligation you have. It is an appreciation that rises up within you for noticing the way that things are. It is a practice of seeing the many ways you are loved, loved by others and loved by Life with a capital *L*. Love comes in many different forms, most of which are not romantic or affectionate in the traditional senses. Love can be a nurse making a special meal request while you're in the hospital; it can be your spouse remembering to take out the trash; it can be a comfortable bed and a fluffy pillow; or it can simply be the energy you have to get up and get dressed in the morning.

When my doctor first suspected that I might have asthma, he ordered an echocardiogram, an ultrasound of the heart, to ensure that my shortness of breath was not caused by an undiagnosed congenital cardiac condition, since that can be common with VACTERL. Thankfully, my heart function is normal. An echocardiogram seems an odd place to find gratitude, but grace lurks in odd places. I was astounded to see my heart beating away on the ultrasound screen. It was working so hard for me without any effort on my part. Again and again it beat steadily to keep me alive. It was so simple and astoundingly profound at the same time. I saw how much I was loved. My body was doing its best to give me an opportunity to experience living.

I don't know anyone who would say that they are grateful for being sick, but there are a myriad of blessings that can come out of illness. There are kindnesses you will see in your family, friends, and even strangers. You will realize that you are stronger than you ever knew. You will see how your body responds to its environment and your moods. You'll ask the big questions and have motivation to follow your most important answers. Little things such as buttered crackers after a surgery or a heating pad when you're in pain will become treasures. You'll feel the healing power of the outdoors, and sense the small victory that is movement. Illness sucks, but life is still pretty dang cool.

The Last Question: What Are You Grateful For?

The last question I asked each woman interviewed in this book was: What are you grateful for? Here are their heartfelt responses.

Meredith

"Niomi. I was told I'd never have kids, and I always said I was meant to be a mom, so Niomi. That's it. There's nothing more than Niomi. I'm so obviously grateful for my family and that I met Gary, but Niomi. She was my gift to Gary because Gary never wanted to be a daddy, and now all he does is tell his friends, 'You have to have a kid. It's the best thing and I never believed it.'

"She's my gift. When I got my wedding dress, I picked out a dress that I think she would probably wear. She's who I'm grateful for. It doesn't get better than that. She makes everyone smile . . . she's my girl. She's me. She's my girl.

"I also have really good parents. I had good parents before this. We're very lucky to have my family."

Sarah

"Definitely my friends and family. And I've got a major Team Wolf support, the type of support that has come out and helped me out. I just went back home to be with my mom for a period of treatment that I'm doing, and she's really helped me a lot. [She is] really supportive.

"We recorded my record because my friends came to my bedroom and recorded me, in my bed . . . singing and playing the guitar and then went away. We did everything else remotely because I can do everything else on the computer. I would listen and tell them what should be done, and we got everybody else to contribute their part—the strings and the bass and the other stuff. It was just this amazing act of generosity and friendship. For that I am super grateful."

Charity

"Oh, my goodness. Even though I said it's not the most important thing, I'm really grateful to be alive, to be able to witness the lives of my mother, my brothers and my sisters, my nieces and my nephews, and all of the wonderful beautiful things that happen in this world. I know that sounds super corny, but I'm not afraid of being super corny. I run around on stage in costumes singing for a living, so corny is not something that is very intimidating to me, but it is such a wonderful thing. I'm so grateful to be able to breathe on my own without oxygen, without a ventilator. I am so grateful. I am so grateful that I can think, 'I'm grateful,' that it is not something I've lost. I'm really grateful to be here to learn and to grow and to love, and that's what I think it's all about."

Lauren

"Oh, everything!—life, family, friends, the health that I do have. I could have a lot worse of a disease. There are people who have it a lot worse with other situations, and I'm lucky that all I have is an autoimmune disease that I can take medication for, or that I can do certain things that can help my symptoms.

"Sometimes I just sit outside and look at a tree, I'm grateful for that tree! It really sounds corny. But sometimes it's just those little things you've got to be grateful for. My food. My house. Everything. I'm blessed in a lot of ways. All the love around me. The people who love and support me. Everybody who's always there for me. I've never been sick in the hospital and not had a hundred relatives there. Everybody wants to come visit and bring something, or do something, and help out, so I'm very blessed in that way."

Kelly

"I'm grateful that I'm alive, and I'm probably most grateful for my children who listen when I go on and on and say, 'This hurts and that hurts and this hurts,' because the list goes on and on. They never say, 'You already told me that' or 'Oh yeah, that hurt yesterday too.' They just listen. Even though they are young people, and they're very busy, most of the time they're concerned about my comfort, and they're a huge help to me. I'm able to do what I do because of them, because of what they were able to give back into my life. I would have been much more comfortable still completely taking care of their lives even though two are in college and two are in high school. I would rather take care of them, much, much rather, but they were perfectly willing to give back to me. One of my daughters travels with me, and she's a full-time college student, but she's also my assistant. She goes with me everywhere I go. She helps me with all my medical appointments, and wherever I go, she's there with me. I couldn't do it if I didn't have her.

"Another thing I can think of: all the patients who give back to me. I get to watch them help each other and give to each other and their community every day, and that's amazing."

Nicole

"I'm grateful for the things that I can still do. I'm grateful for still holding on to much of my cognitive ability.

I'm grateful for my husband. I'm grateful for my support system. I'm grateful for the MS Society. I'm grateful that under all this I'm still able to be myself."

Sharmyn

"Oh my, I am grateful for so many things in my life. I've got to say, one of the things I am so grateful for is that my website has brought so many fabulous women like yourself. I've been approached by some of the most interesting women and men through the Internet, and I'm so grateful that I've met these people. I am so grateful for the doctors in my life who are so extremely brilliant and have compassion for their patients. It gives me hope that we can change medicine because there are a lot [of doctors] who care.

"I am grateful for who I am inside. I'm grateful for who I am on the outside. I am grateful for opportunities that I can see now that I never would have taken before. I'm grateful that I got to do television, I'm grateful that I can just do nothing. One of the greatest things is that I'm just OK being alive. I'm happy to have my life back. I'm secure to do anything. I'm not a hundred percent adventurous to go diving out of airplanes, and that's OK, because it's not a passion of mine. But I am grateful that so many opportunities are out there for people. So many people can make a difference. I am grateful that I see that. I am enthusiastic about life right now. I love that we can wake up and make any decision we want."

Sandra

"Gosh, how much time do you have? There is so much. Life. Life. Life. Of course. That has to be the first thing. And every day that I feel good. And every day that I can wake up in the morning and breathe and can get out of bed and walk around in the world. I am incredibly grateful for my home. My husband is the miracle of my lifetime. I don't know if you read or heard that I married Ron, the Phantom [who performed opposite Sandra in Broadway's *The Phantom of the Opera*], which is crazy. The fact that I met someone who is so supportive and dear to me. I am grateful that my mom is still with me. I am grateful for the father that I had and how his influence continues to inform my everyday life. I could go on and on about my friends and family and the relationships that mean so much to me. I am also really grateful that I have the opportunity to hopefully help other people in some small way. To inspire them to go after their dreams in spite of whatever fears and insecurities they have while, at the same time, letting them know that their happiness, self-worth, and ultimate fulfillment will never come from climbing the ladder. That our challenges really are the path to growth."

Mari

"I am grateful for the opportunity to have this experience in this body. Ultimately, I'm grateful that I have this body because it's my body and mind. I battle with it from time to time, but I am also really grateful when it comes right down to it."

What Am I Grateful For?

I am grateful to be chronically resilient. Each morning I get to start again. I get another chance to be present. More opportunities to live out my values. A new day to tell my husband I love him. Hours to talk to friends and family. Mornings to lounge over tea. Time to become a better student of my health. Minutes to calm my mind. Tomorrow to see things differently. Opportunities to pout and laugh and be sick and be well.

I appreciate my parents immensely. By opening their hearts to me and my challenges, they taught me how to have compassion for my body and accept illness as part of my life. I am thankful for my body. It has been through the wringer and works diligently to support my life. It is my teacher. It pushes me to become a better person. To be more patient, more relaxed, more loving. It reminds me to accept the unacceptable in life. I don't tell it thank you enough, and yet, it does its job day in and day out to the very best of its ability.

And What Are You Grateful For?

Now it's your turn. What are you grateful for? Record your answer in your journal, and if you wish, send me your answer to join a community of chronically resilient readers who rejoice and connect in gratitude. Visit: *www .chronicresilience.com.*

GRATITUDE

What are you grateful for?

EPILOGUE

Sadly, one of our greatest warriors, Meredith Israel Thomas, lost her battle with breast cancer on December 21, 2012. She made the courageous decision to discontinue toxic treatments when they no longer promised to extend her life. From that first estimate of one year to live, Meredith lived more than three and a half. She passed away peacefully holding the hands of those she loved.

During her final months with us, Meredith continued to blog about her experience in the hope that sharing the reality of cancer would create better understanding and urgency around the need for early detection and research. I am overcome with gratitude for her contribution to the book and for being a shining inspiration of how to live fully and gracefully with chronic illness.

APPENDIX A

Values

Abundance	Family	Perseverance
Acceptance	Fearlessness	Philanthropy
Achievement	Freedom	Presence
Adventure	Fun	Relaxation
Balance	Generosity	Reliability
Beauty	Gratitude	Resilience
Belonging	Growth	Respect
Bravery	Guidance	Sacredness
Camaraderie	Health	Sacrifice
Challenge	Honesty	Self-reliance
Change	Humility	Sensuality
Clarity	Humor	Silence
Cleanliness	Imagination	Simplicity
Comfort	Independence	Sincerity
Compassion	Inner Peace	Solitude
Confidence	Inspiration	Spirituality
Connection	Intimacy	Spontaneity
Consciousness	Intuition	Stability
Contribution	Joy	Strength
Courage	Kindness	Teamwork
Creativity	Love	Trust
Curiosity	Loyalty	Truth
Diligence	Mastery	Understanding

Discipline

Discovery

Diversity

Education

Endurance

Entertainment

Expressiveness

Faith

Mindfulness

Money

Openness

Optimism

Order

Originality

Passion

Peace

Uniqueness

Unity

Warmth

Wealth

Wisdom

Youthfulness

APPENDIX B

Financial Resources

Medical Expenses

Medicaid

Medicaid is a government program offered to fund health services for people with limited income. Each state determines its own eligibility requirements. For details visit: *www.healthcare.gov/using-insurance/low-cost-care/medicaid.*

Medicare

Medicare is a government program offered to fund health services for the elderly and certain disabled populations. Medicare Part A pays for hospital stays, home health care, and certain medical supplies. It is offered without any monthly payment. Medicare Part B is called Supplemental Medical Insurance and funds doctor visits, lab tests, diagnostic procedures, dialysis, chemotherapy, and other medical expenses. It does require a monthly premium, although enrollment is optional. To learn about additional coverage options and program details visit: *www.medicare.gov.*

Hill Burton Program

Certain medical facilities are required to provide reduced cost or complimentary services to individuals that meet current Health and Human Services poverty guidelines in return for grants and loans received by the government. To see if you are eligible, visit a Hill Burton–obligated facility and apply through their finance or admissions department. A list of participating facilities can be found at: *www.hrsa.gov/gethealthcare/ affordable/hillburton/facilities.html.*

Pre-existing Condition Insurance Plan (PCIP)

If you have been denied insurance because of a pre-existing condition and you have been uninsured for at least six months, you can purchase health insurance through the state you live in. Premiums, plans, and benefits vary by state. Visit: *www.healthcare.gov/law/features/choices/ pre-existing-condition-insurance-plan/index.html* and click on the state you live in to learn more.

Health Insurance

If you have accepted a new job or if it is open enrollment with your current employer, be sure to look carefully at your health plan options. Check deductibles, co-pays, hospital benefits, prescription coverage, and provider network. Annual deductibles can be quickly met when your health takes an unexpected turn. Your human resources department will be able to help you understand the differences between the plans they offer.

Income Assistance

Social Security Disability Insurance (SSDI)

If you have paid into Social Security and meet certain recent work requirements, you may be eligible for social security disability benefits. Visit: *www.ssa.gov/pgm/ disability.htm* or speak with your Social Security representative for details.

Supplemental Security Income (SSI)

Supplemental Security Income is a benefit designed for people with limited income and resources who are over sixty-five, blind, or disabled. It is not dependent on having paid into Social Security. Visit: *www.ssa.gov/pgm/ssi. htm* or speak with your Social Security representative for details.

Long-Term Disability Insurance

You may have disability insurance as an employee benefit or as a private purchase. Contact your insurance representative or human resources department for details on submitting a disability claim to begin receiving benefits. The amount of your benefit is typically a percentage of your income prior to becoming disabled and may be offset by any Social Security benefits received.

Retirement Plan

If you have a retirement plan in place, many have hardship/disability provisions to avoid a penalty for early withdrawal. Check with your retirement provider for details.

Home Equity Loan

A home equity loan is based on the accrued equity in your home. Contact your bank or mortgage provider to see if you qualify.

Reverse Mortgage

If you are at least sixty-two years old, some mortgage companies will lend on the equity in your home to provide additional monthly income. Check with your mortgage company to see if you qualify.

Places to Look for Donations

- Charitable foundations

- Civic/social welfare organizations

- Churches

- Community groups

- Corporations with charitable giving budgets

- Health associations: go to *www.healthfinder.gov* to search for associations related to your specific diagnosis.

- Friends and family: visit *www.giveforward.com* to set up a web page that friends and family can make donations through.

BIBLIOGRAPHY

ABC News Staff. "100 Million Dieters, $20 Billion: The Weight Loss Industry by the Numbers." *ABC 20-20* (May 8, 2012): *abcnews.go.com*.

Bernhard, Toni. *How to Be Sick: A Buddhist-Inspired Guide for the Chronically Ill and Their Caregivers.* Somerville, MA: Wisdom Publications, 2010.

Boyd, Jeffrey H. *Being Sick Well: Joyful Living Despite Chronic Illness.* Grand Rapids, MI: Baker Books, 2005.

California Department of Transportation. "The San Francisco–Oakland Seismic Safety Projects Corridor Overview." (2012): *baybridgeinfo.org*.

Cooper, Andrea. "The Healing Power of Touch." (2008). Originally published in *Redbook* magazine, retrieved from *www.webmd.com*.

Cooper Marcus, Clare, and Marni Barnes, eds. *Healing Gardens: Therapeutic Benefits and Design Recommendations.* New York: Wiley, 1999.

Doheny, Kathleen. "Nature Has Charms That Can Reduce Stress." *Los Angeles Times,* (July 25, 1989): *articles.latimes.com*.

Dorsey, E. Ray, David Jarjoura, and Gregory W Rutecki. "Influence of Controllable Lifestyle on Recent Trends in Specialty Choice by US Medical Students." *The Journal of the American Medical Association* 290, no. 9 (2003):1173–78.

Edelstein, Julia. "What Women Can't Let Go." *Real Simple* (April 2012): *www.realsimple.com*.

Ehrenreich, Barbara. *Bright-Sided: How Positive Thinking Is Undermining America.* New York: Metropolitan Books, 2009.

Franquemont, Sharon. *You Already Know What to Do: Ten Invitations to the Intuitive Life.* New York: Jeremy P. Tarcher/Putnam, 1999.

Fredrickson, Barbara. *Positivity: Groundbreaking Research Reveals How to Embrace the Hidden Strength of Positive Emotions, Overcome Negativity, and Thrive.* New York: Crown Archetype, 2009.

Fried, Caren S. "Positive Thinking—Helpful or Harmful for Cancer Patients?" *Thoughts on Living with Cancer.* Maywood, NJ: New Beginnings, 1998. *www.cancer-thoughts.com*.

Gawain, Shakti. *Creative Visualization: Use the Power of Your Imagination to Create What You Want in Your Life.* Novato, CA: New World Library, 2002.

Gollwitzer, Peter M., and Gabriele Oettingen. "The Role of Goal Setting and Goal Striving in Medical Adherence." In *Medical Adherence and Aging, Social and Cognitive Perspectives*, edited by D. C. Park and L. L. Liu, 23–47. Washington, DC: American Psychological Association. 2007.

Goodman, Brenda. "The 18-minute Doctor's Appointment Challenge." *Arthritis Today. www.arthritistoday.org.*

Sethi, Ramit. "The Master of Persuasion: Interview with BJ Fogg" *Hustle Your Way to the Top* (January 2011): *www.iwillteachyoutoberich.com.*

Simonton, O. Carl, Reid Henson, and Brenda Hampton. *The Healing Journey.* New York: Bantam Books, 1992.

Kay, Mary. *Miracles Happen: The Life and Timeless Principles of the Founder of Mary Kay Inc.* New York: HarperCollins, 1994.

Kramer, Stacey. "The Best Gift I Ever Survived." TED Talk (February, 2010): *www.ted.com.*

Miller, G. Wayne. *The Work of Human Hands.* New York: Random House, 1993.

Mipham, Sakyong. *Turning the Mind into an Ally.* New York: Riverhead Books, 2003.

Robbins, Mel. "How to Stop Screwing Yourself." Video (June, 2011): *www.youtube.com.*

BBC News. "Self-help Makes You Feel Worse.'" (July, 2009): *news.bbc .co.uk/2/hi/8132857.stm.*

Sloan, Richard P. "A Fighting Spirit Won't Save Your Life." *The New York Times* (January 24, 2011): *www.nytimes.com/2011/01/25/ opinion/25sloan.html.*

"Today's Research on Aging." Population Reference Bureau, no. 17. June, 2009.

Turkle, Sherry. "Connected, but Alone?" TED Talk (June, 2012): *www .ted.com.*

Ware, Bronnie. "Top 5 Regrets of the Dying: A Palliative Care Nurse Shares What She Learned While Caring for Her Patients." *More* (February, 2012): *www.more.com.*

Wood, Joanne, W. Q. Elaine Perunovic, and John W. Lee. "Positive Self-Statements: Power for Some, Peril for Others." *Psychological Science* 2009.